FibromyAWESOME

MELANIE O'SHEA

Cover design: Ultimate World Publishing

Layout and typesetting: Ultimate World Publishing

Editor: Anita Saunders

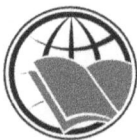

ULTIMATE WORLD
—— PUBLISHING ——

Ultimate World Publishing
Diamond Creek,
Victoria Australia 3089
www.writeabook.com.au

To my beautiful girls, Rhiannon and Isobel, who were my two greatest reasons to heal and get off the couch.

To my amazing husband, Sean, who makes me feel like I can take on the world.

CONTENTS

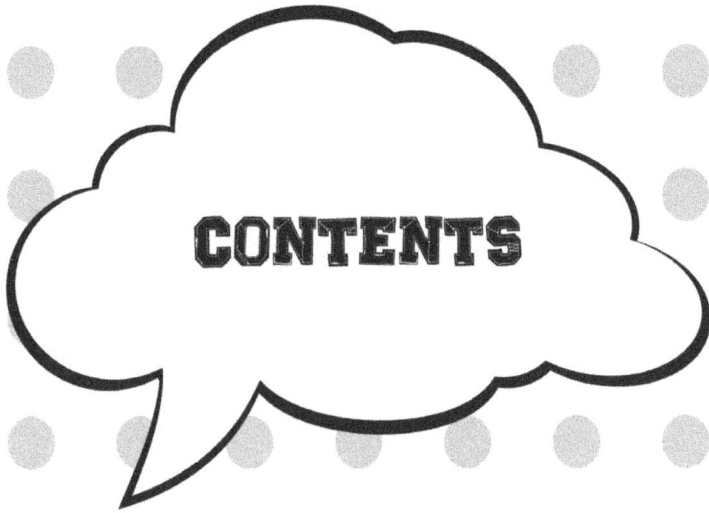

GET YOUR ATTITUDE ON ALREADY!

GET YOUR LIFE BACK FROM FIBROMYALGIA.

Hi, and welcome to my book!

This is a book written especially for anyone with fibromyalgia; there's also a lot of good stuff in here that would help those with chronic fatigue, adrenal fatigue or low immune system. Or anyone worn out, exhausted, overworked, under pressure or just burnt out. This book is for all of you out there who, like me, have spent years doing everything for everyone else, and have put yourselves last, day after day. Now you've used up the last energy reserves in your body, and you're just really struggling to get through day to day.

I wanted to write this book to, first and foremost, give hope for recovery. I know it's something that I wasn't given when I was first diagnosed, and I know through talking to other people that it's still not something that is dished out at the doctor's office when the word fibromyalgia comes up. I wasn't even given options to try, apart from medication. Looking back and seeing how far I've come, it felt important to me to use my experiences to be able to give options to others so they can get themselves better.

At my core, I'm a healer—I want to help others to heal, and I want to see and know that I've helped others to get back to the life they want. I don't believe that a diagnosis of fibromyalgia should stop you from having the life that you want. Hopefully this book will show you that and you'll be able to achieve what you want to achieve. Treat this book as a guide to kick-start your healing from fibromyalgia, or to kick-start your journey towards feeling happier and healthier.

I wanted this to be a book that people can pick up and see that it's not too heavy on the info or the science mumbo jumbo, and is easy to read and follow. The steps are all set out for you here in the book and if you just follow them, you'll hopefully heal a lot faster and make a lot more progress in a shorter period of time than I did when I was going through my own healing journey. I didn't have a book. I just figured it out myself, step by step, so I want this book to give others a much faster way to claw their life back from fibromyalgia.

It was never a dream of mine to write a book. Writing has always been something that I enjoyed, but I never saw myself as an author. It wasn't something I had ever considered until a few months ago. A very good friend of mine told me that a friend of hers had recently been diagnosed with fibromyalgia, and that her friend was feeling really overwhelmed, and had been told what most of us are told—that there wasn't really much she could do about it.

My friend asked if there were any tips that I could give her friend, and I sat down a few nights later at my laptop and wrote about four pages of tips and info in a Word document. It just poured out of me in about 30 minutes. I was quite shocked to see it all in black and white, and to see that I actually do know a lot about healing from fibromyalgia. It was an 'aha' moment, where I realised that I've come a really long way and, just through my own research, and trial and error, I've come through the other side of the tunnel. I sent the pages on to my friend to send on to her friend and I thought, oh my goodness, I could actually write a book about this. I could help so many others, if I could just get my information out there.

That's where the inspiration for this book came from. Since the day I started thinking about writing this book, I've been quite shocked at how many other people have told me that they know somebody with fibromyalgia—their mum, their sister, their friend, or their client.

Seven years on from my own diagnosis, I thought that research would have come up with some options by now, but there really aren't any. Every time I've spoken to somebody about my book, I've been surprised at how many people are out there trying to struggle through without any hope or options put in front of them.

FibromyAWESOME is a condensed guide to the last six to seven years of the healing that I've experienced, and the things that have worked for me; it is your guide to getting started with healing from fibromyalgia. Really, I couldn't imagine not doing this book. It would be selfish of me to not do it! So here it is!

Please be kind to yourself, and take your time getting through FibromyAWESOME. I have written the book in the order that I believe gives you the best chance of success with your recovery, but you can start wherever feels right for you. Each chapter will give you suggestions and a short to-do list; some are going to be harder for you to do than others, and that's okay—every little baby step is getting you closer to the life you want. Doing something is always going to be better than doing nothing!

Try to follow through and complete each step before moving on to the next—you'll feel a lot less overwhelmed if you take it one step at a time, and you'll be in a better head space to see it all the way through.

I know how much everyone is loving affirmations and mantras at the moment, so I've included one at the end of each chapter. Hopefully they'll get your mind thinking healing thoughts (or at least give you a giggle!).

As you're reading through, please connect with me on Facebook @ultimateyoubyyou—let myself and others know how you are healing, and if there are any other tips and suggestions you can offer others. I'd love to hear from all of you, and by sharing your story, you can also help others to recover from fibromyalgia, and together we can reach out and give even more people hope.

I wish every single one of you all the best in getting your life back from fibromyalgia.

It's time to get FibromyAWESOME!

Yours in healing,

Melanie

FOREWORD

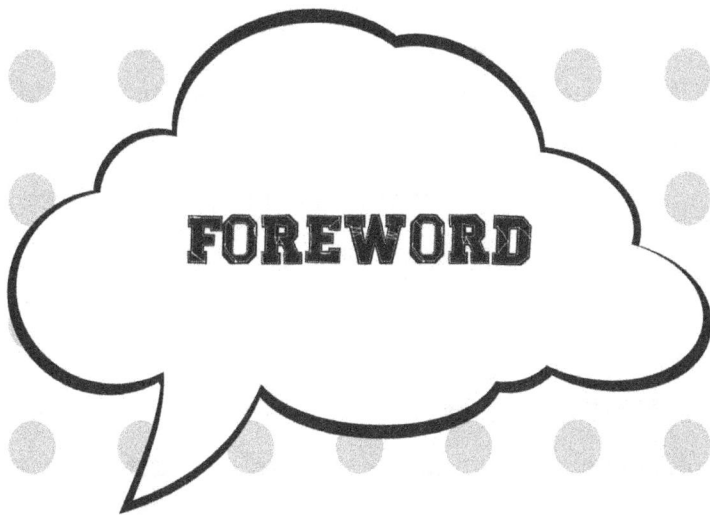

FibromyAWESOME is a valuable resource for anyone who has been diagnosed with fibromyalgia, and doesn't know where to turn.

Melanie's first foray into writing is insightful, humorous, easy to read, and is written in short chapters so as to not overwhelm the reader.

Although Melanie has years of experience healing herself from fibromyalgia, and has worked in the medical field, she doesn't overload the reader with information or scientific words.

Melanie refuses to treat the reader as a victim, and knows the importance of hope and how the reader can change their health by changing their attitude, or mindset.

Melanie tells us to question the treatment options given to us, and to think beyond the medication route. She encourages the reader to drop the labels and beliefs that come from medical practitioners, and from themselves.

As someone diagnosed with fibromyalgia, I have found FibromyAWESOME comforting to read, as well as interesting, insightful, well sourced, and the tips and suggestions are easy to implement.

I have read it many times already!

You won't find any blank pages to fill in, yoga poses, recipes, or an overwhelming amount of advice in Melanie's book, but you will find a wonderful resource that will give you hope and guidance when it comes to dealing with fibromyalgia or any chronic health condition.

Kate Cuzzilla

Teacher/tutor living with fibromyalgia

RAINBOWS AND LOLLIPOPS

Unless you've been living under a rock for the past decade or so, you surely would have heard about the power of a positive mindset to make your life awesome. Don't worry, this isn't going to be a chapter about how you need to spend all day trying to picture yourself running on the beach with a big smile on your face like you're in a tampon ad.

I know how unrealistic it is to make your mind go there when you're lying in bed in agony for the bazillionth day in a row. You've probably already read this sentence three times, but your head is so foggy, nothing is sinking in. Trying to get your mind thinking only positive thoughts at this stage is ridiculously unrealistic—you're just going to stress because you can't make your mind go to your happy place of rainbows and lollipops, and stress and fibro are a bad combo!

At this point in time you don't need to believe your life will one day be just like your happy place, you just need to start to believe that you don't have to spend the rest of your days feeling as crappy as you do right now. After all, change happens when you change your attitude (and mindset is really just a fancy word for attitude!).

If you can just get your head to believe that feeling better is possible, that you may actually one day not feel as lousy as you do now, then you will be able to achieve a massive change in your health. This is really where your recovery starts.

If you can't get your head there, if you can't get your attitude on, and believe that you can feel better, then this book was really a waste of your time and money.

If you can change your attitude, you can open up possibilities for yourself, and you will become more motivated to become better informed. You'll have hope for a better future and that's really the best place for anyone to start. Get your attitude on already!

I remember the day my attitude changed, and now I call it my Attitude Change day—my AC day. It was the day my life changed, because my *attitude changed*. I remember, on this day, being on the couch just absolutely exhausted, just so fatigued, and in so much pain, that I couldn't play with my children. I felt like I was just a lousy mum, like I couldn't be the mum I wanted to be for them.

Every day had been the same for weeks, and I finally decided on this particular day that this was not going to be my life, this was not going to be my kids' life. I'm not going to settle for this life, for being the mum who can't enjoy life with her children. That was when the leaf, so to speak, turned over for me and my healing really began.

Start right here: get it in your head that you need this day, you need your AC day. Don't wait for it to happen, like I did. Just pick a day, put it in your calendar if you have to, put it in your diary, and set a reminder to come up on your phone's calendar, and commit to it. Make a commitment to yourself that that is the day when everything will change for you. That's the day you will start to get your life back from fibromyalgia. It will be the day when you actually start to hope that things can be better.

You need to accept that there are things that you can do to heal from fibro. There are things you can do to have a better life, to get to the life that you want to live, back to the life that you were living before your diagnosis. You need to get it in your head that it actually is a very real possibility, and something that you need to aim for.

And remind yourself that there are people who are living with fibromyalgia—people who are living normal lives, who are working and raising children on their own, or studying and having fulfilling relationships, or writing books. And I'm here, I'm living proof in black and white that it is possible.

For ages, all I could do was Google options for treatment for fibromyalgia. Slowly but surely, I started giving myself options. I started finding options for myself, when no one else could give me any. From there, I found hope. Each day that hope grew and grew, and I've continued over the last seven years to hope.

Now I can look back and know that it all started with my AC day. Without that day, I may still be on the couch. I would have missed so many precious moments with my girls, and they would probably be caring for me by now.

This chapter aims to help you stop believing and stop accepting what you have more than likely been told by doctors, family and friends, and other party poopers: that all you can do now that you've been diagnosed with fibromyalgia is learn to live with it. That's such a load of bollocks. What I really want for you to accept right now is that it is bollocks.

You might be thinking, well, all those doctors and all those specialists, they're really well educated and if they're telling me that there are no treatment options, and no hope of recovery, then surely they would know. To that I would say: for sure, doctors and specialists are very well educated and knowledgeable about surgery and medication and tests; however, they're not really formally educated on alternative treatment options.

As you would know, with fibromyalgia there isn't the option of surgery, nor is there the option to just take tablets and you will feel great, and live a healthy, vibrant life. It doesn't really work like that with fibro.

You need to accept that, yes, there are options with medication, and sometimes people have a real improvement in symptoms from taking the pills. If you want more though, and you don't want to live your life relying on medication, or dealing with the side effects, there are other options for you.

Accepting that you can better your life, heal yourself, and have the energy and focus to really chase the life that you want is one thing; however, you may be thinking, well, this is a chronic, incurable condition. Yes, fibromyalgia may be something you will always live with. That doesn't mean you can't live a satisfying, enjoyable, fulfilling life with it. You don't have to just learn to live with it as you are now. Stop accepting that this is as good as it will get for you.

Many of you may have already tried positive thinking, visualisation, the law of attraction and so on and so forth. Yet, there you are, still on the couch, still in pain, still struggling just to get through every day. You might be thinking, well, what difference does my attitude really make?

For now, try to forget about convincing yourself that your life is going to be all about rainbows and lollipops. Or that one day you're going to be done with fibromyalgia for the rest of your life, and just be an absolute picture of glowing health. At the moment, that's a bit much; it's a bit of a stretch for the ol' noggin. For now, just work on believing that your health and your life don't have to stay the same as they are now, or worse.

For the moment, that's as far as you need to take your mind. Your AC day is a great way to kick-start that change in attitude. Your AC day will signify the moment when you started to take back control over your own health, when the clouds began to clear a little. It is a day to celebrate! So, make sure you put it on your calendar now, if you haven't already, and commit to making the day happen.

Share your big day with others; make it a big deal with your family, connect with people on Facebook, or in forum groups. You could start your own forum group and encourage others to share their AC day! Connect with me on my Facebook page (www.facebook.com/ultimateyoubyyou), or in my Facebook group—'Positively FibromyAWESOME'—or email me (hello@ ultimateyoubyyou.com) and let me know that that's your day. I'd love to see how different people celebrate their AC day!

I don't want you to expect that after your AC day, your mindset will stay in that great place of acceptance and hope each and every day. I can keep my attitude in check now—even on the 'bumpy' days when walking over a molehill feels like climbing up a mountain (not that I've ever come across a single molehill, but you get what I'm saying)—but it wasn't always that way.

For a long time, I struggled a lot with my mindset, and I saw every day when I didn't feel as fabulous as I thought I should as evidence that I was failing to get anywhere. Now I just see those days as a gentle reminder from my body that I need to make time for myself to relax and recharge my batteries, and I put that time in my schedule for the day. I also use that time to reflect on where I have come from, and where I am heading—it helps put things in perspective.

You will have days where you find it really hard to believe that you have made any real progress, or ever will—the perfect time for a little reflection! Keeping a journal will make it easy to reflect and will give you real evidence of your progress. Your AC day is a fantastic time to begin writing.

Write about how you are feeling on that day, how it feels to believe that you have begun moving towards the life that you want, and how it feels to know that you don't have to give up on your dreams simply because you were diagnosed with fibromyalgia.

Journal on the good days and the bad days. When you have those days when self-doubt is messing with your mojo, you will be able to read back through your entries and remind yourself of how far you have come, and why it is so important for you to keep dusting yourself off each time you trip over a molehill.

Well, here you are—you have nearly finished a chapter of a book! Go, you! I remember how hard that used to be for me. I would fall asleep after a paragraph or two, and maybe not have the energy to try again for a day or two, and by then I would have forgotten what I'd already read.

I've really tried to keep this book as short and easy to read as possible, but don't worry if it takes you a while to get through it. For now, just skim briefly through the book. Don't try and implement too much. Just have a bit of a look through, read some bits and pieces that you think might be most relevant to you.

Try to really understand and accept how far I've come from where I started with fibromyalgia to where I am now, and try to convince your mind that you too can improve. If it's possible for me it's possible for you. Believe it!

In the introduction I promised you an affirmation for each chapter, so your affirmation for this chapter is: *My life won't be all rainbows and lollipops but it will be AWESOME.* Say it again and again until you believe it!

WHO'S IN CHARGE?

Growing up with a mum who was an old-school, hospital-trained nurse I understood that doctors knew all. You get sick, you go to the doctor, they give you tablets or cut you open and (hallelujah!) you get better.

Fast forward a decade or two, I was diagnosed with fibromyalgia, and by a specialist doctor, no less. I was told that the general consensus within the medical profession was that there really wasn't much to be done about it. I could dope myself up with a combination of painkillers, antidepressants and anti-anxiety meds, and, basically, I'd just have to learn to live with it.

I was given a life sentence with no chance of parole. Huh? Really? I pay you $400 and that's the best you've got? It didn't sit well with me, but my mum trained me well (bless her) and I knew that what the doctor says goes.

That is, until my AC day. Lying there on the couch with my little cherubs parked in front of the TV, I did something that I had never really done before—I considered that the medical profession might be wrong.

Maybe, just maybe, they didn't know everything. Maybe, I didn't need to accept this as my new normal for the rest of my days. So, I Googled. I Googled whenever I could manage it, which was only a few minutes at a time back then.

Gradually, I found myself treatment options. I put myself in charge of my recovery and my health and, day by day, I've gotten my life back. In fact, I'd say my life is now even better than it was before fibro!

One of the best things about putting myself in charge of my recovery was that I finally had hope, when the medical profession couldn't give me hope of ever improving my symptoms. I was able to set goals for myself, and I started to think about a future where I could achieve what I wanted to, be the mum I wanted to be, to have the life I wanted to have.

When you put yourself in charge of your health, you get to do fibromyalgia the way you want to. *You* determine how you approach your symptoms, and your recovery. *You* determine how you progress, *you* set the pace, and *you* make the changes when you're ready.

You'll become more informed about fibromyalgia and about treatment options, about what other people have done. That means you'll be better equipped to educate your family, friends, boss, whoever, and that means you'll have a more understanding support system around you.

You will also find yourself better able to manage flare-ups—you will know what works for you. You will have tools in your belt, and you will know when and how to use your tools to get through flare-ups the quickest way.

Once you're in charge of your health, you'll feel more confident. Your self-esteem will skyrocket, your mood and general outlook on life will be sunnier, and you may even feel more in charge of other areas of your life. You could end up with a life even better than it was before fibro, like I have!

Once I put myself in charge of my health, I found that I had the confidence to not only tackle single parenthood, but also a nursing degree. It had been about two decades since I'd been at university and here I was, looking at studying again—not only was I in a bad way with fibromyalgia, but I had two young children who depended on me. I wouldn't have even considered taking on all of that if I hadn't re-energised my confidence by putting myself in charge of my health; it was a real turning point for me.

Once I felt in control of my health, once I felt like I had some say in what went on in my body, I developed this urge to look at other areas of my life and take inspired action. I can tell you that that is an amazing feeling to have. I found that one small change led to many more, which led to even more; it triggered a beautiful cascade of re-jigging and improving my life. So much better than accepting status quo!

Now, just a few years later, I'm a published author! To put yourself and your experiences out into the world in a 'self-help' book takes a lot of confidence. A heck of a lot of confidence! Pre-AC day Melanie O'Shea certainly didn't have the confidence to even think about writing a book, let alone actually make it happen!

Once you know within yourself that you have a say in your health, your mind will perceive situations differently. You will see opportunities and challenges, and you will want to grab them by the horns and steer them in the direction you want to go.

On the other hand, if you never take charge, and you leave yourself without options, nothing much is going to improve for you in your life. You will continue to be just another fibromyalgia sufferer, playing the victim card, and saying goodbye to your dreams.

You can choose to sit back and wait for your doctor to fly in your window with a beautiful bright cape, and some new miracle drug—or you can choose to be your own hero, and *save yourself*.

Start by educating yourself. Read this book (obviously) and then, if you haven't already, get on Google, see what you can find out about fibromyalgia. What's the consensus about the causes? Is there a consensus? What about the triggers and the risk factors? What are the treatment options? Is there anything you haven't already tried that I haven't covered in this book? You really need to know this yourself.

Don't rely on doctors or other people to tell you what your options are. Don't rely on this book to give you all of the information either. I don't claim to know everything about fibromyalgia, and I'm still looking every day for new things that I can try. Just because I feel my health is in a great place now, doesn't mean it can't get even better!

When you're in the thick of fibromyalgia, it's overwhelming to think about taking charge of your health, especially if you've never considered yourself as having any say at all.

Just thinking about where to start with your recovery is probably enough to make your head feel like it's going to explode. Hence this book! Ta-da! This book will give you the steps to get out of the fibro fog that is seeping into every area of your life—it will give you the jump-start you need to get going again.

When reading this book, I recommend working on one chapter at a time, but you may prefer to start with the one thing that you think would make the biggest difference to your life, or the one thing that would be the easiest for you to get moving on.

Wherever you start making changes, make sure you stick with one thing until you think you've got a pretty good handle on it, then move on to the next easiest or most important, or the next chapter, and go from there.

Although you will be in charge of your health, it's very important that you don't discount what your doctor has to say. I'm my mother's daughter, and I do have a lot of respect for doctors. I do think that if you find the right one, they can be very valuable on this journey towards recovery.

At the same time, don't be afraid to ask your doctor questions, or to disagree with their treatment plan. Ask for a second opinion if you're not satisfied with what your doctor tells you. Don't be afraid to say I found this on Google or my friend told me about this, or I read about this in a forum; I want to try this, or I want to discuss this. That's okay, and even if that's all you do at the moment in terms of taking charge of your health, then that's an awesome place to start.

If the message isn't getting through, stamp your feet and say, it's my health, it's my body, I want to know what my options are, I want to know why you want me to do this or why you don't want me to do that. I want to know! Don't let them pressure you into anything that you are not comfortable with, or make you feel that you have no right to question what they say.

You don't need to know the research or the science behind everything that your doctor suggests, but it's your body, your life, your health, and you have every right to know where their opinion is coming from.

You might be thinking, I'm just too tired, my head's really foggy, and I just can't sit through a spiel from my doctor, or take in all of this information, or stamp my feet. I get that, I really do. Like I said, when I started out, I could only do a few minutes at a time reading websites, and that was it. My brain was just mush. But that's why you've got this book.

I've made this book intentionally easier to read, easier to implement. Just start here, and at least have a conversation with your doctor around wanting to know your options. And if they can't give you any, tell them you'll find your own, and you hope that you have their full support.

You may have actually had times before where you've said to the doctor, look, I don't want the meds—maybe they weren't working for you, you felt they weren't right for you and so you stopped taking them. Then you ended up with a massive flare-up and now you're feeling a bit scared about not having the medication or not having that as an option. Or maybe you're doing really well on medication and you don't see the point in not having them. You're travelling along okay and you don't feel the need to try anything else. I would wonder why you bought this book if that were the case!

I've got absolutely nothing against taking medication. In fact, as a nurse, I have a good knowledge base about the role of medication in health. I'm not saying pills are evil and you should flush them all down the toilet right now. All I'm saying is, you are in charge. If part of you being in charge of your own health is saying I make the choice to take this medication, then that's a great place to start.

Having said that, there's no reason why you can't be on medication and still try other options (as long as you first check with your doctor about how those changes might interfere with your medication). You may even get to the point where you're feeling pretty good, and you find that you're ready to start weaning off the medication (please, please don't ever stop taking medication suddenly without chatting to your doctor first!). There may come a time when you don't need the medication at all. How great would that be?

At some point in your life, you may have had an experience with a health professional who really doesn't appreciate that the patient has the right to question them, or to have any say in their own health. It's certainly a situation I have come across in the past. I've questioned a doctor or made a suggestion regarding something I had read, and the response from the doctor was almost as though they patted me on the head, and said you don't need to worry yourself about that, dear, just follow doctor's orders and you'll be fine.

My response to that is I just don't go back. I find a doctor who is willing to listen to my opinion, and to encourage me to try options that feel right to me. If you find yourself in a similar situation— where you've done your research and you want to explore your options, and your doctor pats you on the head—just remember back to your AC day.

Remember that day when you decided to believe that you can get better, and remind yourself that you don't need your doctor's permission to do so. You don't need your doctor to make it happen for you, to say it's okay to make your own choices. You're in charge, not them! You've made the decision to get better— don't let anyone take that away from you.

Start talking about your plans for recovery to other people— family, friends, colleagues. Speak as though you are the CEO of your health—you are the boss, and whatever you say goes. Talking to other people about the options and information you have found will build your confidence, it will help you to feel that you are actually in charge of your health. You will show others that you know your body well, and you know what's best for your body. Saying it all out loud will help you believe that you've got this.

If bragging about your plans to become fibromyAWESOME isn't really your thing, then get your journal out. Write to yourself about how awesome you are, and how the decisions that you've made, and are going to make, are going to get you to a healthier, happier place. Give yourself a pat on the back, and refer back to that when you're feeling a bit low in confidence. It will remind you that you have taken charge of your own health, and no one can take that from you unless you let them.

Your affirmation for this chapter is: *I am the all-powerful CEO of (Your Name) Health Inc. I am in charge and what I say goes.*

FIST PUMPS

Madame CEO, before we go any further, we need to address the issue of your team. Your newfound position of CEO of (Your Name) Health Inc. requires you to build a team of worthy individuals who will respect you as the woman in charge, and will support and encourage you as you need.

By building your awesome crew you can lighten the load on yourself, which is going to reduce the stress in your life, and give you more time to focus on your healing. With less pressure on your time and body, and more time to focus on you, you'll be able to achieve results faster—that means feeling better sooner! And who doesn't want that?

First on your fist-pump crew should include family and friends who are understanding if you need to cancel social outings, who will pick up the slack with babysitting, housework, grocery shopping, and mani-pedis (okay, that one might be pushing your luck a little, but it never hurts to ask!). I actually wish, looking back now, that I'd reached out to my family and friends a lot sooner after my diagnosis than I did. I was a big believer in being independent and going it alone. I guess I wanted to prove to myself and everyone else that I could do it all.

Asking for help is something I still struggle with, and it's only been the last couple of years that I've really allowed myself to do so. I think it's pretty safe to say that I would have gotten to where I am now a lot faster if I had leaned on my loved ones more, if I had just let them help me. There were plenty willing to, but I was too proud to accept that I needed their help.

I really didn't do myself any favours, and I made getting to where I am so much harder for myself. I want you guys to get there sooner, so please, just reach out, just tap into any resources that you can. It is literally going to save you so much pain. Just bite the bullet, swallow your pride, and admit that you could use some help.

Once you've done that, the next hurdle is to tell them how they can help you. This is something I find even harder to do than admitting that I need help. Don't be afraid to assign jobs to people. Send out an email or a Facebook message each week or month, and say these are the things I really need help with at the moment, and who wants to do what? If your loved ones have put up their hand to help you, trust me, they want to know the best way to do that.

If you don't have family and friends who are nearby, and can physically help you, (and even if you do) having a supportive and encouraging crew available by phone or Skype, or even email, is just as important. You can always pay for somebody to do the cleaning or laundry for you. Or pay a babysitter or nanny if you don't have family and friends who can give you a break from the kiddies, or book the little ones into childcare or crèche, and the school-aged into after-school care a couple of days a week.

You can still lighten the load if you don't have family and friends nearby, you'll just need to pay for it. If you can't afford to pay for it all, pick one or two that you can afford, or that place the biggest physical strain on you, and budget for those.

As well as reducing the physical stress on your body while you heal, you're going to need plenty of emotional support and encouragement. You've got to put good people around you who are going to give you perspective—remind you of where you're going, and where you're coming from. They're going to help you on those days when you feel that you're getting absolutely nowhere.

The best people for this job are your cheerleaders. You need cheerleaders who are going to say, look at what you're doing, you're doing amazing, you've come so far, keep going; they will wave pom poms in your face and help you get up on the lousy days and stay focused on moving forward. Cheerleaders will remind you that you have hope when you feel like giving up— they are important people to have on your team.

A good cheerleader will not only be able to spell out your name, but will infect you with their positivity, and they will feel comfortable with pulling you back to reality when you try to build those molehills into mountains. We all need someone who cares about us, and empathises with us, but is not afraid to tell us to stop being a drama queen when we need it.

Next on your team should be your trusty doctor. Like I spoke about in the previous chapter, make sure your doctor believes that you are capable of healing from fibromyalgia, and is okay with you calling the shots and wanting to discuss any or all aspects of your care. If you are taking medication for fibromyalgia, or want to explore your options with medication, make sure your doctor has experience prescribing those medications for fibromyalgia.

If you are in the market for a doctor, it pays to do your research. Ask around for recommendations for doctors who are open-minded, preferably with experience treating fibromyalgia. Set up some appointments and interview the potential candidates. Tell them this is where I'm at, and this is where I want to get to.

Show them some information and options that you've found, and see how they respond. See if they're encouraging and supportive of you bringing in ideas and if they respect you as CEO of (Your Name) Health Inc. If they're not open to discussing your options, or you feel they won't respect you as being the one in charge of your health, then move on to the next one.

If available to you, go for a doctor who specialises in integrative medicine (IM), and you'll get more bang for your buck—a doctor with knowledge and experience treating conditions with not only medication, but also nutrition, supplements, lifestyle changes, and possibly alternative medicines (acupuncture and the like). You basically get a bunch of healthcare folks in one well-rounded team member.

I found a fantastic IM doctor about a year ago, through a recommendation. I hadn't even known about IM doctors before that, but I wish I had. I wish that I'd been able to tap into his brain and his resources a lot earlier. Although I was already in a pretty great place with my health before I met him, he has helped me to tweak some areas, and I'm amazed at the progress that I've made in the last year.

As you go through this book, you might need to add more allied health people to your team—exercise physiologists, counsellors, etc. Once again, make sure that you do your research and find team members who are open-minded, have experience treating fibro, and will tailor an individual program based on your input. Just remember, you are the almighty CEO and you are in charge, regardless of who you accept into your crew.

You want all of the healthcare people on your team, and not just your doctor, to be willing to listen and discuss treatment options that you've found through your research. They should also be constantly on the lookout for breakthroughs that can help their clients. You don't want people who have been doing the same old thing for 20 years, and aren't interested in introducing anything new into their practice.

The best healthcare team members will have your best interests in mind, and will help you weigh up the risks and benefits of your options. They will also appreciate that you ultimately decide which path to take.

You also need to know that your doctor and other healthcare team members are watching your general health. Don't forget there's fibromyalgia and then there's your overall health. Fibro is just one small piece in the overall picture of how well your body is handling life.

I don't know if you know, but having one chronic condition actually gives you good odds for getting another one. I'm not a betting woman, because I hate spending my money on things that I have no control over. The odds of me developing another chronic condition though ... I'd put money on that, because I know I now have control over those odds.

I might have been a higher risk of developing type 2 diabetes, fatty liver disease, high blood pressure, even heart disease at one point—when I spent most days barely moving off the couch, my cells were stressed out all of the time, and my diet, when I did manage to eat, wasn't much better than the cookie monster's.

Now, though, I am not at any greater risk than any other woman my age; in fact, I'd say I have a lower-than-average chance of developing another chronic disease, probably even lower than when I was in my 20s! My blood pressure and heart rate are great, my weight is in a very healthy range for my height, my cholesterol and triglyceride levels (amount of fatty guys, called lipids, in the blood) are fantastically low, and I'm the fittest and happiest that I've been in a very long time.

I digress ... Yes, because you have fibromyalgia, you are at a higher risk of developing further chronic conditions, but do not accept that that will happen. It does not have to happen; you control the odds here. It's very important that your team doctor is keeping an eye on things, like your cholesterol, blood pressure, and vitamin and mineral levels, and not just focusing on fibromyalgia.

Hopefully this chapter will help you to start putting together your team, to build an offensive against fibromyalgia as a solid unit. If you can swallow your pride and take the time to build a supportive, encouraging, helpful, educated, open-minded crew to start with, you'll give yourself a great kick-start towards becoming fibromyAWESOME.

Repeat after me: *Fist pumps for me. I have an awesome crew who will back me up whenever I need.*

LOSE THE CAPE

Forewarning—You might not like what I have to say in this chapter. I may receive some less-than-glowing feedback from it, which will be good, because at least I'll know you've read it.

I live a sugar-free life, so there won't be any sugary coatings of any description here. Just try to keep an open mind and trust me when I say that I wish someone had told me this years ago. You are not Superwoman, you will never be Superwoman. You are human. Just lose the bloody cape already. Untie the strangling bright red ribbon around your neck and just breathe.

The people of Earth will be just fine if you drop the act and reveal your vulnerable, worn-out, exhausted, overworked, underappreciated and imperfectly perfect humanness.

Owning at least some of the responsibility for the position that (Your Name) Health Inc. is now in is part of being CEO, and you won't do yourself any good trying to throw someone else under the bus. You're in charge of what happens to (Your Name) Health Inc., remember?

Maybe you've been told by your doctor that your fibromyalgia came about because of a virus. Maybe that's true, but that doesn't mean that you have no responsibility for ending up where you are now—maybe if your immune system wasn't so beaten down by you not taking care of yourself for so long, the virus wouldn't have had such a lasting impact. Maybe it would have just been a virus that came and went in a couple of days and didn't turn into a chronic condition.

If you now believe that you have the power to heal yourself (and if you don't, go back to the first chapter and start again!) and recover from fibro, you also need to believe that you have the power to keep your health as it is by sticking with the status quo.

Maybe you're a stay-at-home mum who spends your days planning the perfect meals, and running your kids around to a dozen different extra-curricular activities every week (because perfect mums don't say no to their kids, right?). Maybe you're working 60 hours a week and working on a PhD at the same time. Maybe you're running your own successful business, and doing the work of three people by yourself. Maybe you just can't feel content unless every single thing in your life is perfectly organised and planned out for the next 20 years.

I can own a couple of those. Can you? If you're reading this book, I'm guessing you can, or something very similar to those. Well, guess what—it needs to stop now.

In case you missed my subtle point, here it is reworded: you will not recover and live the life you want if you cannot admit to yourself that what you have been doing has not worked for you, drop the Superwoman act and accept that you are an incredible, amazing, powerful and inspiring being who matters to people simply because you are you. Phew, that was a mouthful!

Now is the time to leave your superhero standards at the door, and trust that the universe won't implode if you do. If you can do that, you will be able to focus on getting better, which means you will recover faster. Isn't that worth accepting that less than perfect is perfectly okay?

It's time to create new standards for yourself. More realistic, more acceptable, human standards. If you can get your standards to a more reasonable place, then you're going to find that you are better able to prevent flare-ups, and any flare-ups that you do have will be less nasty. You're actually going to be able to put more energy into the enjoyable moments in your life. Isn't that why we're all here?

I was listening to a podcast a little while ago, and I had this 'aha' moment and things just clicked; it was just simply the phrase 'perfection doesn't exist'. Even though I'd heard it before, and I'd said it to myself many times, all of a sudden it just clicked. Perfection does not exist.

Since then, it's been so much easier for me to accept that I don't need to be perfect; I don't need to expect everyone around me to be perfect; I don't need to have the perfectly cleaned house; I don't need to have the perfectly written book. I can get things done without them being perfect, and that is my new standard.

The good-enough standard—that's what I aim for now. It is such a weight off! Perfection doesn't exist—consider that a bonus affirmation for this chapter, and repeat it to yourself until you believe it!

Dropping the superhero act is not something that comes easily for me though; I have always been a high achiever, and aimed for perfection in everything I did, and hated on myself when I couldn't get there. At the moment, I'm going through a process of blending two families into one household.

For the first time in a very long time, I have another adult in the house who, bless him, wants to help out with cleaning and mowing, and running the kids around town, and picking up groceries, and so on. He's fantastic, and I am truly grateful to have someone willing to share the load, but it's also the cause of so much frustration for me.

I'm used to living a pretty organised life with my girls and feeling like I had a lot of control over what happened and didn't happen, and how everything happened. Now there's another adult in the house, and I can't control everything anymore. The way I did things for years when it was just myself and my girls doesn't really work now that there are two extra people coming and going, and some days I feel so unorganised I feel like my head is going to explode. It's been a massive struggle for me to give up some of that organisation and control.

I'm not going to tell you that it's easy to change your ways. Like me, you may have always had high standards for yourself. That's not a bad thing, but expecting yourself to always live up to those standards is contributing to fibromyalgia taking over your life.

When I was studying nursing, I wasn't happy with just passing, I had to get high distinctions, and I would get cranky at myself if I didn't get them. If I got 95% for an assessment, I would be disappointed that I didn't do better. That's where my expectation was for myself, and I made myself sick trying to be the perfect single mum uni student. Looking back now, remembering the toll that my high standards had on my health, I feel quite ridiculous that I placed a higher priority on my grades than I did on my health.

You've got to take some ownership over what happens now, and stop blaming your doctor for not having the answers, or your husband for not helping out enough at home, or your boss for relying on you so much.

If you can't accept any responsibility for where your health is now, and you can't bring yourself to lower your standards from superhero to human, then your recovery from fibromyalgia is going to be more difficult and more drawn-out than it needs to be.

Not to mention those nasty old flare-ups—you may not notice much improvement at all, and if you continue to think that perfection is the only way to go, and keep pushing yourself to get there, chances are you're going to get hit with flare-ups more often, and they'll become more and more severe. I really don't want that for you; I want you to start making some progress, and to get to the point where your life is whatever you want it to be as soon as possible. I want you to have a life that you design for yourself, not a life that is determined by fibro symptoms.

You might be thinking, well, hang on, it's a bit unfair to say that I've gotten myself here; I shouldn't be feeling bad because I've got high standards in life. Of course not. I do not think that there is anything wrong with having high standards for yourself, I think high standards are important for us to succeed and to achieve what we want.

At the moment, though, the only area of your life where you should be aiming high is your health. In fact, for your health, I encourage you to aim for the highest possible standard you can imagine right now. For everything else, until you get your health back on track, you want to be aiming for good enough. Accept that you are an imperfectly perfect human.

Your affirmation for this chapter is: *I am not a superhero, but I'm still totally awesome.*

TRIM THE FAT

Hands up if you're sick of hearing about how you need to manage the stress in your life better? Yep, I hear you. If people want me to stress less, they should stop telling me to stress less. Stop stressing me out about stressing out!

So, I apologise in advance for this: you need to stop stressing so much already.

I can imagine you glaring at the page right now and thinking this book was a big fat waste of your time and money. Just hear me out for a minute. I do know that if it were as easy as 'just stress less', you probably wouldn't need to read this book.

It's ridiculous to expect you to become Zen like a Buddhist monk. However, the fact of the matter is, if you want to reclaim your life from fibromyalgia, you need to reduce the physical and emotional stress bombarding your body. It's time to trim some of the fat from your life. I'm talking about toxic relationships, ridiculous work hours, coaching your kids' sports teams, drama-filled friendships.

While it's true that nobody knows for sure what causes fibromyalgia, the general consensus from everything I have read about it is that stress seems to play a significant role in its development and in triggering flare-ups. I know I had had way too much stress in my life for way too long, and I think I may have had fibro, with mild flare-ups, for years before it was actually diagnosed. When I separated from my then-husband I think it was the straw that broke the camel's back, and my body just couldn't handle any more stress, and that's when fibro really hit with full force.

Most of us have been taught by our parents that it's wrong to be selfish, and that we should always be thinking about the needs of others. These are messages we tend to carry into our adult lives. For a long time I acted like I was the saviour of those around me, and I've put a lot of pressure on myself to try to fix everything for my dearest and nearest.

I put myself last on my to-do list for such a long time, and ran myself into the ground because I felt that doing everything I could for others made me a good person; it's a familiar pattern I still slip into at times. I have to remind myself that I'm actually being selfish when I'm trying to make myself feel better by accomplishing everything, and aiming to be awarded the Most Awesome Woman Ever trophy.

I know now when I need to take a step back and chill out—I get what I call mini flare-ups. I will feel the fatigue first, then my legs or my head will start to ache, my energy levels dip and so does my motivation.

There is no doubt in my mind that physical and emotional stress are fibro triggers for me, and if I try to push through, my symptoms will get worse, and instead of recovering in a few hours, it will take me a day or two to recover. I don't want that, so I try to pick chilling out over pushing through as much as possible. Like I talked about in the last chapter, it's about taking responsibility for your health.

Maybe you are running yourself into the ground because you don't want to let your husband down, or you can't say no to your kids, or maybe you feel your boss and colleagues can't possibly manage without you. Maybe you've enrolled in university, or taken on extra hours at work, or you've gotten yourself voted in as president of the school community, or just launched your own business.

Now you refuse to admit you can't do it all, because you're not a quitter, and people are relying on you. Come on, admit it—you know deep down you're making yourself sick with your incessant need to prove to the world how strong and selfless and truly incredible you are, because you can do anything you put your mind to. Well, I say pfft to that.

Do you need someone to tell you it's okay to drop the balls, cancel appointments, pull the kids out of sports, resign from your presidential duties, or drop your hours at work? Or break off a toxic friendship or a relationship that you've already been in way too long? Do you need someone to tell you that you it's okay to trim the unhealthy fat from your life, so that you can give yourself a fighting chance to heal and actually have the life that you want? No problem, here it is.

You do not need to do it all. Just say no. It is okay if you are the number one priority in your life.

Now read it again. And again. Read it as many times as you need to until you believe it, then go and get rid of that fat.

You get rid of the fat, you get rid of the stress. You're going to sleep better and have less fatigue. You're going to have less pain, and migraines, and you're going to have more energy. (How good does more energy sound right about now?) You can have better moods and less of those horrible, depressing mood swings and miserable days. Less brain fog—you'll be able to have clearer thinking. Heck, you might even be able to read the rest of this book!

I'm not saying that you can't be there for other people, but at the moment you have got to be number one. It may take time for you to be okay with that—old habits die hard, after all.

My eldest daughter, Rhiannon (12), has a rare genetic disorder called Williams Syndrome, and my youngest, Isobel (10), has dyslexia, which makes learning very difficult for her. Up until halfway through this year, I had spent years taking my girls to countless therapy and medical appointments, and tutoring, and any activities that I thought might help them. I exhausted myself with the constant running around, and the pressure I put on myself to try to 'fix' them.

This year, I reached the point where I said I'm done; I need a couple of afternoons a week with nothing on after school, and more time to do what I want to do. And then came the guilt. Wow, talk about mummy guilt!

It was difficult for me to be okay with putting myself first for a change, but I kept telling myself that I'll be a better mum if I take care of myself first, I will help my kids more if I'm a little selfish, and my girls will be happier. Turns out I was right! My girls have thrived, and we enjoy our time together more now. Who knew you can be a better mum if you take care of yourself first!

I moved on from the guilt and you need to be able to do that too. You need to accept that trimming some of the fat from your life and putting yourself at the top of your to-do list is the best thing for you and your family.

Think about it: you will be making yourself well, so you will be in a much better position—with loads of energy and a clear head—to be helpful and supportive. Now, don't take that as me saying that you need to make yourself better so you can help more people—that's the kind of thinking that got you into this mess in the first place! I'm simply saying you have got to help yourself before you can help anyone else.

It's like the oxygen mask demonstration on planes—how can you expect to assist others to put their masks on if you suffocate? You've got to put your mask on first, fill your lungs, and only then can you save your fellow passengers!

You probably feel really selfish at the moment, just picturing putting yourself first, but you've got to change that attitude—being a good, selfless person doesn't mean doing everything for everyone and putting yourself last all of the time. Realistically, by trying to do everything for everyone else, you're actually being more selfish.

You probably feel that so many people rely on you for so much—kids, elderly relatives, your boss and colleagues, clients, the whole school community—that you're in a position where you can't afford to drop the ball at all. I know the feeling well.

The question you need to ask yourself is: can you afford to not drop the ball?

Look at where you are. You're absolutely no good to anybody in the state you are in—unwell with the flare-ups and fatigue and pain, and lying on the couch or barely getting around, or maybe unable to even get out of bed at all most days. Are you really able to juggle everything now anyway?

All of us have some areas in our lives where it really doesn't matter if you drop the ball a little bit. Does it really matter if your seven-year-old kid misses a soccer training session or ballet class now and then? Is it really going to affect them or their future prospects that much? I'm sure even the most elite professional athletes around the world missed a few training sessions when they were kids! You can certainly lower the amount of time and energy that you're putting into some things in your life, and everyone will be just fine.

There were times when I was at university, going through my nursing degree, when I had to accept that I couldn't manage everything. There were semesters when Rhiannon had been really ill, or something had happened within the family, or I had enrolled in too many units over Christmas/summer semester, and the stress was piling on thick. There were semesters when I had to withdraw from one or two units, and I even had to withdraw from a whole semester a couple of times.

I wanted to get through my degree as quickly as possible, so it was always frustrating when I had to withdraw, but now that I've finished uni and been out a couple of years, I actually don't know why I was in such a rush. I put a lot of unnecessary pressure on myself, and created so much extra stress in my life, and I paid the price with my health time and again.

When I did finish university, I got a graduate nurse job at my local hospital, and they are not easy to come by in my region. I thought, I'm so lucky to be here, I can finally earn some good money while helping people, and I can totally do the nursing thing and the single mum thing at the same time.

I am awesome and I can do it all. How quickly I had forgotten the flare-ups from trying to do it all while I was at uni!

There was so much stress from my job and from trying to stay on top of everything at home as well that it didn't take me long to burn out big time, and I started getting nasty flare-ups again.

Then I got really sick with the flu, and for weeks and weeks I struggled to recover, but I kept on pushing through. In the end, I had to quit my job that I had worked so hard to get. It was one of the hardest decisions I had to make, and quitting is not something I do easily, but I had no choice. I just couldn't risk my health anymore—I had two kids who needed me, and I didn't want to go back to living my life on the couch.

In the end, it took me months to get back to where I was before I started working, and I have no doubt that I'd be struggling to get out of bed each day by now if I'd stayed in my job. I am hopeful of picking up some casual nursing work soon, but I have my wonderful man Sean to help me out now, and I will only work as much as my body can handle. I have no desire to go backwards with my health again!

An easy way to get into the habit of changing your priorities is the trusty to-do list—who doesn't love them! I've always loved my to-do lists, but my list would end up being a page long, and it would be so overwhelming that I wouldn't really get anywhere with it, and I never seemed to have time to do things for myself, like exercise or meditate.

Now I have a max of five things on my to-do list at a time. That's it; I don't put any more on it until I've crossed some off. And I don't start on my list until I've eaten well and exercised—my health is at the top of my list.

So, what are the four most important things you need to get done today, plus at least one thing for yourself?

You may also be able to trim some stress from your life by having a good hard look at your relationships and friendships. Are there friendships in your life that are completely one-sided, that are all about you being there for them, but when you're needing help they're not there for you? Are they just somebody that needs to rant and rave to you about all the problems in their lives? It's one thing to be a friend, but at the same time you can't take on everybody else's stress and drama, and expect that it won't affect you.

Maybe you're in a relationship that you know is not good for you; it's not worth the drama, but you feel like you owe it to the other person to stick it out for another month, which then becomes another year. Every day you're in that relationship or friendship you're adding stress to your life that you really don't need.

Remember, stress is one of the biggest triggers for flare-ups. If you want to do anything about making yourself better, then you've really got to be a little bit ruthless with the stress and the drama, and even the people, that you allow into your life.

It's important to trim as much fat from your life as you can, but obviously we can't expect to have completely stress-free lives, unless we want to join the Tibetan monks. You've got to find some way of getting your body and your mind to chill out, so you can deal with the unavoidable stress. For you, that might be meditation or guided visualisations, or bubble baths, or even hypnosis.

I had my first experience with hypnosis about 18 months ago and it was amazing. I wish I had done it sooner. Hypnosis helped me so much with my anxiety and it really helped me to gain some perspective on the stressors in my life, and the ability to deal with the stress a lot better. I can't recommend it enough.

If you can't see somebody in person for hypnosis, or if that's not something you're comfortable doing, then there are some really great apps, YouTube videos, and audio files on the internet where you can actually practise some self-hypnosis, or you can get specialised recordings to help you deal with particular issues, like anxiety.

Otherwise, start making meditation, or guided visualisation, a part of your daily routine. I prefer to do it at night before bed, but some like to start the day with meditation. You might think that you don't have time for it; start with five minutes at a time, just give yourself five minutes.

Everybody can give themselves five minutes a day to chill out and shut off and just focus on yourself; five minutes is nothing. Then you will actually find that those five minutes become so sacred to you that you will want more, and it will become easy to increase that to 10 minutes, or 15 minutes. You'll start to feel the benefits, and soon you will find that you'll want to make time for it.

So, to sum up, stress and fibromyalgia don't mix. If you won't trim some of the fat from your life, if you're determined to keep pushing through, your flare-ups are going to continue. You might as well accept that where you're at now is where you're going to stay.

Or, you can decide that your health is more important, and start cutting the crap, the day-to-day drama, the stress where you can, and make yourself your number-one priority. So, trim as much stress from your life as you can, and get into the habit of meditating, or something else that's going to help you get through the times when you can't control how much stress is in your life.

Your affirmation for this chapter is: *It's all about me, me, me and that's how it should be.*

HAD A GUTFUL

Here's a little something for you to digest. The general consensus in the world of medical and healthcare types is that if our guts aren't healthy, we aren't healthy. Now sink your teeth into this little morsel: food is medicine. Let that sit and ferment with you for a bit. On the table in front of every single one of us is the power to make a very real difference to our health, simply by changing what we eat.

Now, to be clear from the start—I am not a dietitian. I'm not claiming to be an expert on food and digestion matters. I did do a subject on nutrition during my nursing degree, and I have read a lot about nutrition in my quest to heal from fibromyalgia, but I am by no means qualified to tell people what they should and shouldn't be eating, and that is absolutely not my intention with this chapter.

I will share with you what has worked for me, and I would encourage you to also try similar changes to your diet, but only after you've checked in with a qualified dietitian. Dietitians have completed at least an undergraduate degree, and are experts on nutrition and diet, and treating medical conditions through diet.

Just like trimming the fat from your life, tweaking your diet will help you to experience less pain and inflammation in your body. You'll be able to sleep better, and have more energy and less fatigue during the day. You'll actually find that your muscle strength can improve, and you'll have less muscle fatigue. You'll be boosting your immune system, and you'll be less likely to catch all the bugs going around (and we all know how getting sick can trigger a fibromyalgia flare-up).

Now I know, nobody wants to have the realisation that they have to give up the things that they love, especially when it comes to their diet, in order to improve their health. We all want to keep doing what we're doing, because change is hard, and changing our eating habits is super hard.

Just give us the quick-fix option already!

The truth of it is, though, if you're not willing to tweak your diet at all, if you're not willing to experiment with removing certain foods from your diet, you're probably going to struggle to see any real change in your symptoms. We really are what we eat—if you continue to eat the same, expect to continue to feel the same.

You may not know it, but there could be a whole host of underlying issues going on in your body contributing to your fibromyalgia symptoms. Some of those issues could be the result of an unhealthy digestive system. Our digestive systems can become damaged over the years due to the use of antibiotics and other medications, poor diets, lack of exercise, and illness. This damage may be on a microscopic level, but it can have a massive impact on our health.

Essentially, unhealthy gut equals unhealthy person. Fortunately, it's also true that if we can make our guts healthier, we'll feel healthier. You still may not want to hear it, but it needs to be said—one of the best places to start is often with our diet.

In my experience, some of the biggest dietary triggers for inflammation and fibromyalgia symptoms are gluten, dairy, sugar, alcohol, and caffeine. I've also briefly read about some new research around red meat causing inflammation in some people. I've never really eaten a lot of red meat, but I have reduced my meat intake and started having one or two meat-free days a week, and I have noticed that my digestion seems less sluggish, and my energy levels slightly higher on those days.

Now, before you start panicking and thinking that you're going to have to survive for the rest of your life on rice and water if you want to heal, hear me out. You don't need to be extreme with your diet changes, and I'm not saying that you'll never be able to eat the food that you love again.

I certainly didn't wake up one day and decide I was going to cut out 90% of the foods from my diet. I cut out one at a time. Well, I actually started with completely removing dairy and gluten, but I hadn't been eating much of either for a couple of years already, since doing an elimination diet, under the guidance of a dietitian, pre-fibromyalgia.

I'd highly recommend going through an elimination diet with a dietitian—you might be surprised to find how many of your symptoms can be managed better simply by changing what you eat. If you can't afford to see a dietitian, then you can actually access elimination diets on the internet now, and there are books that will walk you through a whole elimination diet.

If you can't access a dietitian, I'd recommend at least checking in with your doctor before you start cutting foods out, to make sure that you're not at risk of developing any vitamin or mineral deficiencies, and to check that dietary changes won't affect your medication dosages—changing your gut health and weight loss may affect how your body digests certain medications, and how much you need to take.

During the elimination diet, I discovered that gluten was responsible for the chronic back pain and knee pain that I had had for years as a young adult. After only a couple of days without gluten, all of my pain was gone, and then it was back again within a couple of hours of reintroducing gluten into my diet—it was quite incredible!

I eat a little bit of gluten now and then, but if I eat too much, I'll feel it within a few hours. My digestion gets sluggish, I bloat, my back aches, my legs and knees hurt, and my energy will be low.

If I really overindulge in gluten I'll just be an absolute mess the next day. It's like overnight dementia—I can't think straight, my head is so foggy I have trouble concentrating, and even holding a conversation is a struggle, because I have so much trouble getting the right words out, and I feel so fatigued and flat. Knowing all that will follow if I do, it really makes me rethink ordering a bowl of pasta.

The elimination diet also showed me that dairy is a no-no for me. Dairy tends to hit my head—headaches, fatigue, heavy-headedness, dizziness and pressure in my sinuses.

I very rarely have any dairy at all anymore. I have almond and coconut milk in my tea, and there are a lot more options available now for yoghurt and cheese alternatives. I actually really like coconut yoghurt, and I've recently discovered a creamy dairy-free feta that Sean and I both love in our breakfast omelettes.

Once I got more serious about reducing the amount of gluten and dairy in my diet, I was ready to tackle sugar. Through my early fibromyalgia Googling days, I had come across information that said sugar was a major cause of inflammation, fatigue, muscle pain, migraines in many people. Sound familiar? I figured if eating sugar could be responsible for some of my symptoms, surely I was better off without it.

It took me a couple of goes to actually quit it completely, and to keep it out of my diet. When I did, though, and got past the awful withdrawals, I knew it was one of the best things I'd ever done for my health. I noticed I was getting a lot fewer headaches and migraines, and less muscle pain; I was sleeping better, and had loads more energy throughout the day; my moods levelled out and stopped swinging all over the place.

Even my menstrual cycle has been affected by my sugar-free lifestyle—I don't really have PMS to speak of, apart from being a little irritable and headachy for a couple of days, and I don't really get period pain much at all anymore. Just a little bonus for giving up sugar. Oh, and I lost about a kilogram a week for the first eight weeks! I wasn't even exercising at the time!

Even though I still have cravings for sugar at times, I will never eat it again. It's just not worth it. New Year's Day 2019 marked four years since I quit sugar cold turkey; four years since I've had refined sugar in cakes and biscuits, or soft drink, or lollies and chocolate. Yep, four years! I'll pause here for your applause ...

Thank you, thank you! It's a huge accomplishment for me; I wasn't a part-time, treat-myself-to-two-squares-of-dark-chocolate-once-a-week kind of sugar consumer. I was seriously addicted. It wasn't something I could just eat in moderation. If I ate some, I'd eat more, I'd eat it all—that was my approach to sugar for many years, and I still have to be very careful.

Last year, I was very sick with vestibular migraines, and I believe they were brought on by the amount of sweet 'sugar-free' treats I was eating—bliss balls, slices, and raw chocolate sweetened with refined sugar alternatives like dried fruit, rice malt syrup, coconut nectar, etc.

Although I still wasn't eating refined sugar, I had gradually increased the amount of 'healthy' sugars in my diet (the more sweet food I eat, the more I want—classic addiction behaviour!), and in excess, any form of sugar is obviously bad for my health, so I try to avoid it all, bar one to two pieces of fresh fruit a day.

I don't drink alcohol anymore either. Up until a few years ago, I was able to tolerate the occasional drink with dinner. Now, if I have even one drink, within an hour or so my legs ache, my head is heavy, and I need to go home and go to bed.

Recently on holidays on the beautiful Sunshine Coast of Queensland, with Sean and our girls, we stopped in at a tavern for lunch. It was a gorgeous Queensland summer day, the first day of our holiday; the sun was shining and the sky was blue, and everyone was in such a great mood.

I really felt like a drink with lunch, so I ordered a half-nip of Bacardi with soda water and fresh lime. I only got about halfway through my drink before I felt so tired all I wanted to do was go back to our holiday house and nap. And that's how I spent the first afternoon of our holiday, despite plans to spend it at the beach. I won't make that mistake again.

If you do want to indulge, try to choose a low-sugar option—white spirits are usually a good option, with soda or sparkling water and a lime or lemon wedge, rather than soft drink. Beer, wine, and cocktails are best avoided as much as possible.

I know I sound like the Fun Police. Friends and family actually joke about how my diet is gluten free, dairy free, sugar free, and fun free—they think they're hilarious. I think they're just jealous because they see how awesome I am and how great I feel!

I will admit, though, initially, it wasn't easy to deny myself so many of the foods that I love, especially during social occasions, when it seemed like everyone else was eating cake or drinking alcohol. But then I figured, at least I was able to socialise—something that didn't happen much at all when I was having nasty fibro symptoms all of the time.

I always have people telling me life is too short to deny myself chocolate or 'real' pasta, but I tell them life's too short to spend it on the couch in pain.

Now, if you've ever looked at the gluten/dairy/sugar-free foods at the supermarkets or at the specialty shops and cafes, you probably would have seen that they're pretty expensive, and you might be thinking that there's no way you can afford a gluten/dairy/sugar-free life.

Luckily, you don't need to go out and buy a bunch of those products. In fact, the cheapest, and best way to cut those foods out of your diet is to just eat more fresh, whole foods. You know, the stuff that doesn't come in packets. As a bonus, you'll also cut down on the amount of salt in your diet, and other artificial bits and pieces that aren't good for you, and you're probably going to find that you actually save money, because you're not buying a heap of packaged rubbish.

Now that I've freaked you out by telling you I had to give up all the yummy food to feel better, I'm going to give you some good news. A really easy thing that you can do for your health, without making any major changes in your lifestyle, is to just drink more water.

Chronic mild dehydration, which is where you're not quite drinking enough water on a regular basis, can actually cause symptoms like brain fog, fatigue and muscle pain. I know if I've had a day where I haven't had enough water, because I'll wake up in the middle of the night with leg cramps.

If you're somebody who, like me, habitually struggles to remember to drink enough water, then there are actually some really handy apps that can help you. I have been using an app on my phone that notifies me when it's time to drink some water, and I can set the timeframe between reminders. The app also tells me how much water I should be drinking each day, based on my weight and age, and if I record each drink, it will let me know whether I'm on track to reaching my target intake. You've got to love technology!

This chapter has covered a lot of information, and I know that thinking about changing your diet as much as I have changed mine could be overwhelming.

I want to point out that I didn't cut gluten, dairy, sugar, and alcohol out of my diet all at once, it was a gradual process that I did as I was ready. If you're really not ready to face the possibility of life without chocolate and soft, fluffy bread, I would highly recommend that you at least reduce your sugar and alcohol intake, and work on drinking more water each day—at least it's a start.

I can still go to Italy one day, even if I can't eat anything there is your affirmation for this chapter.

BLOODY HELL

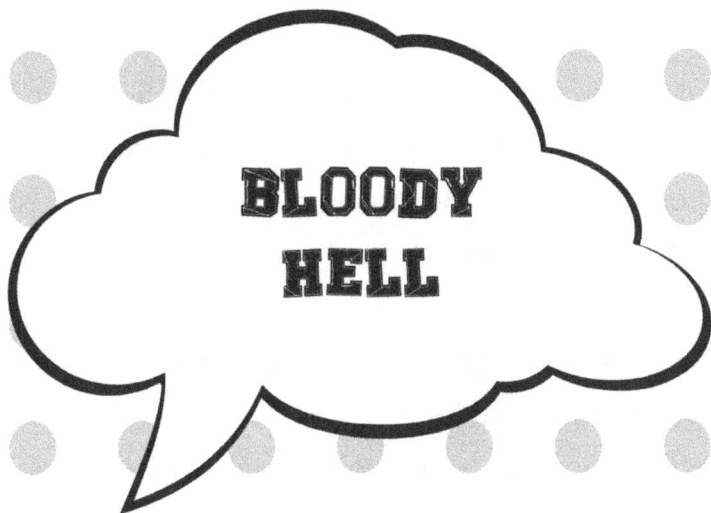

I'm quite sure the last thing you feel like doing at the moment is being more active. More than likely, you're struggling just to get out of bed every day. Your body is probably screaming at you already, and moving it more than absolutely necessary seems plain ludicrous. I get that, I really do.

Unfortunately, you have to get the blood flowing if you want to give fibromyalgia a kick up the bum. You need to start moving more. Yes, that means the 'e' word: exercise. Sorry for the foul language, but it had to be said.

You're probably thinking *Bloody hell, woman, are you insane?* right now and that's okay. I'm sure it's not the first time someone has thought that of me. However, there's really no way around it. Your head is telling you that the last thing you need is to move more, but it's so full of fog it can't be trusted. So, trust me—my head is clear. If it makes you feel any better, you don't need to worry about exercise at the moment. In fact, you can just forget about that word for now.

What you really need, what your body is craving, is movement. That's what you need to focus on for now—just get moving, and get your blood flowing. Your blood cells want to get around your body quickly to do their jobs, and your muscles and joints want to be able to fulfil their purpose in life. Don't you want that for them? Of course you do!

It's not all bad news though. Massage is also a great way to get your blood flowing like it needs to. And to help your muscles and joints do what they need to do. Yep, I just gave you an excuse to book in for regular massage. Rejoice! I bet you're feeling a lot more love for me now. I knew you'd come crawling back. Try walking next time, it's good for your legs.

The really good news is that once you start moving, and getting massages regularly, you'll find you have less muscle tension, which means less muscle and joint pain, and quicker recovery from flare-ups. Yay! Hopefully, in time, this will lead to you being less reliant on your pain medication. Plus, less pain generally equals more good-quality sleep. And what happens when we start sleeping better? That's right—more energy during the day, improved mood, less brain fog, and generally feeling better than when our sleep quality is lousy.

So, do you need to start training for marathons and climbing up mountains to feel better? Nope! Do you need to start pumping weights and doing a hundred sit-ups a day? Nuh uh!

The absolute worst thing you can do for yourself is push yourself to go from couch to buff and fit as quickly as you can. It became obvious to me pretty early on that the harder I pushed myself the slower my progress.

You see, fibromyalgia is a stubborn cow—the more you try to push her forward, the more she'll dig in her hooves and refuse to budge, or she'll start backing up on you. To get movement in the right direction, you need to gently coax her to take small, slow steps forward, when she's ready.

Not long after my Attitude Change day, I started trying to exercise. A lot of the reading I had done about fibro said that regular light exercise was super important for managing the symptoms. Part of me was hoping it wasn't true, because it was truly the last thing I felt like doing—it seemed like the opposite of what my body needed. My body told me every day that I needed to rest and sleep more. But I was willing to try anything and everything if it meant a better life for myself and my girls.

When I was first started trying to exercise with fibromyalgia, I struggled just walking slowly on a treadmill for more than a couple of minutes. If I tried to vacuum for more than a couple of minutes, the room would actually start spinning, and I would feel so exhausted.

My efforts were rewarded with feeling more fatigued and with more pain than before I tried to exercise, and it would take me a few days to a couple of weeks (maybe even months) to get up the courage to try again. Because I tried to do too much too soon, and was so sporadic with my exercise, I found it didn't get any easier for a long time.

Now, I work out at least five days a week, for 15 – 40 minutes a day, depending on how I feel, and that's in addition to other incidental exercise, like housework, gardening or playing with the kids. And I actually love how I feel after a workout now—I have more energy and I feel more relaxed. I do get sore muscles and feel tired some days, but it's no different to anyone else who works out and feels it the next day. It means I've pushed my body just enough to build a little more muscle, and to increase my fitness a touch.

I get a great feeling of accomplishment every time, and it feels amazing to know that every day I am a little stronger, and a little fitter. I crave exercise if I skip it for more than a couple of days; my body craves it. I never thought those words would come from me!

The real turning point for me was when my Emmett therapist (more on Emmett therapy soon) reminded me that it's much better to make slow progress and be able to maintain it, than to push myself too hard and fast, and end up hurting myself and going backwards more than forwards. She said it was much better to gradually build up the intensity of my workouts, and then maintain that intensity for a few weeks, than to push hard for a short period and then have to go backwards in intensity because of injury or fibro flare-ups.

Although she didn't really tell me anything that I didn't already know, hearing it from someone else made it easier to accept. It's like she gave me permission to take it easy. That day was the start of regular exercise for me, and I made it my mission to just do some form of movement most days of the week, even if it's just a few minutes of stretching. I've maintained regular exercise for months now, and I've slowly, but consistently, made progress. Mission not-so-impossible!

With every week of regular exercise, I find that everyday tasks and activities become easier and easier for me to complete. Things that used to take me ages to do, or would leave me feeling a bit worn out, I now breeze through.

Each day, I pick the type, length and intensity of my workout based on how my body is feeling; I usually manage one or two cardio workouts a week, two or three strength or toning (Pilates, yoga) workouts, and one or two flexibility or stretching sessions.

In late February of this year I joined a touch football team. I played touch throughout most of my teenage years and early twenties, but then I hadn't played for about thirteen years. The first two or three weeks were hard—I was only able to stay on the field for about three or four minutes at a time before I needed a breather, and I felt so sore and tired the day after a game or training session.

Each week, though, I'm able to run around on the field more, with less pain and fatigue the next day. It's such an amazing feeling to go back to something that I enjoy so much, and to know that it's possible because I've worked hard to take my life back from fibromyalgia.

You can't expect to pick up where you left off pre-fibro though, and you shouldn't be aiming for that right off the bat, because you'll be setting yourself up to fail. If all you can do to start with is five minutes of stretching or yoga, or five squats, or if all you can manage is to walk around your lounge room three times, then that's better than nothing.

It's really important to gradually build the intensity and the duration of exercise and, once you get to a point where it feels easy, and you're able to exercise around that level most days of the week without your fibro symptoms getting worse, I would recommend that you stay at that point for at least three to four weeks.

Be able to easily maintain where you're at before you try to do more. I guarantee that if you go too hard, too fast, you will crash and burn, and end up being too scared, too sore, or too tired to move. You will go backwards, and you really don't want to do that. It's so much better to take five slow steps forward than to take two leaps forward and then three steps back.

There are days when I feel like I just can't be bothered exercising, because I'm tired, or I have too much else to get done that day, or I might be having a mini flare-up (usually if I've had a lot going on for a couple of days of the week, or if I haven't slept well, or if I've been travelling). On those days I may only do 10 minutes of stretching or light yoga, but I will feel so much better for it.

It's as though I can actually feel my blood is circulating better; I feel the fatigue lift, and I feel more energised. You don't need to do cardio every day, or feel the muscles burn; if all you can manage is stretching, then that's absolutely better than doing nothing.

A lesson that I learnt the hard way (and I had to learn it more than once before I accepted it), is to be really careful of the days when you feel good. I find that those are the days when I can push myself a little too hard and then I pay for it the next day.

Enjoy your good days, and be grateful for them, but don't overdo it—that extra five minutes on the treadmill today could come back to bite you in the butt tomorrow, and maybe the next day too. You're more likely to skip exercising on the days that follow, and you could lose a ton of momentum (and motivation!).

Maybe you're still not convinced that more movement is going to be good for you. Maybe the thought of improving your fibro symptoms isn't motivating enough. That's understandable; at the moment your foggy head is telling you that moving is bad, and rest is good, and I know how hard it is to ignore that.

As we covered in Chapter 3, once you've been diagnosed with one chronic disease or condition, like fibromyalgia, you are automatically at a higher risk of developing other chronic diseases, like diabetes or heart disease. One of the reasons being if you have a chronic condition or disease, you are more likely to be unable or unwilling to exercise regularly.

You see, exercise is not only good for improving fibro symptoms, but it also helps you live a longer, healthier life! You have just got to get up and start moving—trust me now and thank me later!

Maybe you're still worried that any extra movement will only make your pain and fatigue worse. Just remember, you only need to start slow, and gradually build up your strength and endurance. And making movement a regular part of your routine doesn't need to break the bank either.

You don't need to join a gym or sign up for boot camp (oh, please, don't sign up for boot camp until you are really ready—fast and hard really doesn't work for fibro). You can start by looking up YouTube for some light stretching or yoga workouts, or just walk around your house for a few minutes.

There are some really great websites now with heaps of free workouts, where you can choose the intensity and length of the workout. I love fitnessblender.com; I've been using it for most of my workouts for around two years now, and I can always find a workout that suits how I'm feeling.

You might be thinking you couldn't possibly find time for movement. Well, I'm calling BS on that. Everyone can find five minutes each day to walk around their lounge! And once you can find five minutes, you'll soon find you can spare 10 minutes, 15 minutes, etc. etc. If you need to, schedule in time for movement and write it in your diary, put a reminder on your phone, write it on the family calendar.

You've absolutely got to make time, and this goes back to what I harped on about in earlier chapters—you need to start to put yourself first if you want to recover, reclaim your life and be there for the people you love.

As mentioned above, something else that you need to make time for is massage. Some people with fibromyalgia will find that massages actually make their pain worse if the massage is too deep, so it's important to find a massage therapist who is experienced in chronic pain conditions, and you need to make sure they don't go digging their elbows into your muscles. Massage is great for improving your blood circulation, and clearing areas of inflammation.

Some people just don't like massage; I'm not a big fan myself. I don't actually find massage that relaxing; however, I love Emmett therapy (see, I told you I'd get back to Emmett therapy). My doctor recommended Emmett therapy to me, and I'm glad I gave it a go. It is a really gentle muscle release therapy and I've found a treatment usually only takes around 15 – 20 minutes—not much time to schedule for at all, really.

I can have a couple of niggly areas treated in one appointment, and feel pretty good the next day. I find it relaxes me a lot more than massage too! I haven't tried Bowen therapy—which is another type of muscle therapy—but I've had people tell me it's quite a good option for very light manipulation without increasing or setting off pain, so you might want to give it a go.

If you're worried about the cost of massage therapy, or you can't physically get to a clinic, there are plenty of videos on YouTube, and instructions on other websites, to teach you how to massage yourself. Self-massage is great because you can target the areas where you feel you need it, and then control the depth and the intensity of the massage. And you can do it whenever you need to!

I would recommend using a magnesium cream or gel with self-massage. Magnesium is absolutely fabulous for sore muscles, and you'll notice even better results.

The longer you wait to get moving, and give your muscles the attention they need, the harder it's going to be when you do start. Every day that you stay on the couch you lose a little more of your muscle tone and condition, which means your muscles will fatigue more easily when you do use them, and that makes movement so much harder.

Not only that, you're not going to make as much progress in improving your pain or your other symptoms, and so you'll need to keep chugging down those pain meds, and dealing with severe flare-ups. I don't want that for you, and I'm sure you don't want that for yourself. So, please, get moving and book in for a massage now!

Your affirmation for this chapter is: *Crawl first, worry about running later.*

LIKE A BABY

If you've ever had a baby, the phrase 'sleep like a baby' probably conjures up images in your mind of pacing your hallway for hours on end, with a baby screaming in your ear, or 20-minute catnaps, 24 hours a day, or driving laps around your neighbourhood at 1 a.m. while your baby sleeps in the car.

Generally, babies are pretty lousy sleepers, right? For those first few weeks, especially, they usually have their circadian rhythm all mixed up. They want to sleep all day and keep you awake all night.

When my fibromyalgia was at its worst, I slept like a newborn—I couldn't get enough sleep during the day, but at night, no matter how exhausted I felt, I just couldn't get decent, deep slumber. I'd wake up feeling like I had been running all night, feeling like I hadn't slept at all.

I really had no endurance to get through the day—I would be struggling by mid-morning—and usually, by the time it got to six or seven o'clock at night, I would be so exhausted, I wouldn't be able to sit up to eat dinner. Every day I felt like that, and it was so draining, so depressing.

If you've got the same problem, I've got great news for you—it is possible, and relatively easy, to change your sleep cycle around. When you do, you will find that you actually need to sleep less during the day. You'll be getting good-quality sleep at night, when you're supposed to, and you'll wake up feeling a lot more refreshed, with less fatigue throughout the day.

You will find it will be easier to tick things off your to-do list, and to get through each day without falling in a heap. As a bonus, once you feel you're getting on top of that fatigue, you'll have more motivation, which means you're going to be more likely to exercise regularly, and to eat well (reread the two last chapters if you've already forgotten how important your diet and regular exercise is!).

But wait! There is more good news. Well, not really news, we all know it—the more deep slumber we have, the better our moods. We all know how irritable or emotional we can get when we're tired, and it makes it that much harder to deal with pain, anxiety and depression, if we have any or all of those going on.

When we get plenty of quality sleep on a regular basis, everything seems just a little bit brighter, the intensity of pain decreases, and things generally bother us less.

Until about a year ago, I really struggled to get enough good-quality sleep. I had trouble getting to sleep before midnight, and I had a lot of trouble staying asleep all night. Despite being at a point where my fibro symptoms were pretty well under control, come 6 a.m., my girls would wake me up, and it would be such an effort to get up and get going for the day. Then, come 3 p.m., I'd have a massive mid-afternoon energy slump, and some days I could barely keep my eyes open all afternoon, until around 9 p.m., when I'd suddenly be wide awake and ready to take on the world.

Now, I kind of sleep like a coma patient—I have no trouble falling asleep most nights, and once I'm asleep I stay asleep (with the exception of interference from cats and children). Just about every day I wake up ready to face the day. I'm still not the best morning person, but I don't have to drag myself out of bed, and I don't need two hours to get going in the morning, just my breakfast omelette and a cup of tea. It's a fantastic feeling when you can wake up in the morning, and know that you have a full day of feeling pretty good, and getting stuff done.

I used to waste so much of every day sleeping, but now I very rarely need to sleep at all during the day. There might be the odd occasion when life has been a bit more chaotic than usual for a few days, or if I've been woken up by something (kids, cats, storms, etc.) during the night, or if I'm sick, and I might need to have a bit of a power nap. Those days are rare though, and rather than needing to sleep hours a day, 10 – 15 minutes is usually enough to keep me going for the rest of the day.

Just a bit more information about the circadian rhythm (and it's nothing to do with cicadas, those noisy little bugs that can keep you awake all night). The circadian rhythm is a 24-hour internal clock for your sleep/wake cycle—regular periods of sleepiness and alertness. And it's actually what is to blame for those afternoon or post-lunch slumps, where you just feel like crawling into bed and having a nap.

The circadian rhythm should follow a nice regular rhythm of sleepiness in the evening and then throughout the night, and being awake and alert throughout the day. When you're getting plenty of good-quality sleep at night, those slumps throughout the day will be a lot less noticeable than they are now.

Without all of the scientific mumbo jumbo, all you really need to know is that a lot of brain business, hormones and signals throughout the body contribute to the circadian rhythm working properly, and one of the most important hormones is melatonin.

Melatonin is a hormone released by the pineal gland in the brain. The pineal gland releases more melatonin when it gets dark, and that's a signal to the body that it's time to wind down and get ready for sleep—it essentially helps to regulate the circadian rhythm.

Most people, if they're getting good-quality sleep, should have a sleep cycle that goes for about 90 – 120 minutes—a cycle of falling asleep where your heart rate slows, then the delta stage of sleep, which is really deep, restful sleep when your body makes repairs, and builds and replaces bits and pieces, and then you have REM (rapid eye movement) sleep, or the dream state.

If our sleep cycle is on track, then we shouldn't be getting a lot of daytime fatigue, or massive slumps in energy. Sounds pretty important, right? Yep? So, what you need to do is start getting back on track, and stop sleeping like a newborn (sleeping all day and then struggling to sleep properly at night).

You might be thinking, if I don't sleep during the day, I get so exhausted that I can't do what I need to do to look after my family or my kids. I don't recommend completely cutting out daytime sleep cold turkey, especially if you're at the point of still needing quite a lot of sleep during the day. Getting your circadian rhythm back on track will take time, and you need to gradually cut down your daytime sleep by retraining your mind and body.

Each time you get to the point where you really feel like you need a nap, hold off an extra 10 minutes. Do what you can to stay awake—drink water, walk around the room, weed the garden, put on some loud music.

Try not to rely on caffeine to stay awake though—it will mess with your cycle even more. Did you know that caffeine works by interrupting signals in the brain that tell you that you feel tired? The signals in your fibro brain are already messed up enough when it comes to feeling tired—you really don't want to make the situation any worse up in there!

Once you've been able to consistently wait an extra 10 minutes before each nap, for about a week, try waiting an extra 15 minutes for a week, then 20 minutes, and so on. By gradually reducing your daytime sleep, you'll go a long way towards resetting your circadian rhythm, and having a much healthier sleep cycle—your body will start to adjust to less daytime sleep, and you should notice that you're sleeping better at night.

If you find that despite cutting back your daytime sleep slowly you're still having a bad mid-afternoon slump, try eating a protein-rich snack or smoothie—I find a handful of nuts or seeds, or blending some up with a banana, cacao powder, maca powder and coconut water gives me a nice energy boost that will keep me going until bedtime. Also, make sure you're on track with your water intake for the day—even mild dehydration can have a significant effect on how fatigued you feel.

While reducing your daytime sleep is important for resetting your circadian rhythm, having a consistent sleep and wake-up time is just as important. For most people, any sleep you get before midnight is the most valuable for the body. I have always been a night owl—I would have so much energy late at night, and I'd really struggle to wind down enough to sleep before midnight most nights—and I would miss hours of valuable sleep a week.

I needed a little help to get to sleep earlier. I went to my doctor and said I need to be getting to sleep earlier and getting more of that quality sleep, but I'm so used to going to sleep late that even if I try to go to sleep earlier I don't fall asleep until around the same time anyway.

My eldest daughter, Rhiannon, was prescribed melatonin a few years ago, to help her go to sleep quicker—because she has Williams Syndrome, she also has ADHD and anxiety, and it would take an hour or two (felt like five hours to me!) each night after I'd tucked her in before her mind would slow down enough for her to go to sleep.

I asked my doctor if he could prescribe slow-release melatonin for me, and it has made such a huge difference—I rarely have any trouble getting to sleep around 10.30 p.m. now, and I usually sleep soundly all night (until Rhiannon wakes me up at 6 a.m).

So now, if I'm asleep by 10.30 p.m. most nights, rather than midnight, I'm getting roughly 10 extra hours of sleep every week, while still getting up at 6 a.m. each day. I can tell you, those extra 10 hours make a huge difference!

I wake up in the morning feeling like I've had a great sleep, and feeling like I can get through the day easily. Although taking melatonin helped me, I also had to change my night-time routine to make sure I'm not staying up and getting involved in TV shows or working on the computer late at night when my body should be getting ready for sleep.

Small changes in my routine helped me to gradually make my bedtime earlier. You can't expect to go from trying to get to sleep at midnight to getting to sleep at 9 o'clock overnight; it's not going to happen. Each day or two, try to get into bed 15 minutes earlier—start winding down earlier, logging out of Facebook, and turning off the TV or laptop earlier.

If you find that it's really difficult for your mind and body to switch off and relax before bedtime, then try yoga, stretching or meditation/guided visualisation at night. You could even try a hot bath or self-massage—you'll not only be helping yourself to relax, you'll also be helping reduce pain before bed.

Maintaining regular exercise has also made a big difference to me being able to consistently fall asleep earlier. Exercising during the day helps regulate the circadian rhythm. I know that on the nights where I've done a workout during the day, and I've meditated before bed, I sleep so much better than when I haven't exercised or meditated.

Even if you've done everything you can to fall asleep at a reasonable time, your efforts will be in vain if you are in pain. Pain can make it really difficult to fall asleep, and to get into the deep, restorative phase of the sleep cycle, which is ironic, because without that deep sleep, it's very hard for the body to repair itself, and to manage inflammation in the body. It's a vicious cycle—the less quality sleep you get, the more pain and inflammation you end up with.

On those nights when my pain was bad, I would try to have a hot shower or bath before bed, and it would help to ease some of the muscle tension. Epsom salts are really great for muscle pain—try a handful in the bath, with a few drops of peppermint and lavender oils. Peppermint oil also helps to relieve muscle tension, and lavender oil is relaxing.

After your bath or shower is a fantastic time for a little self-massage with some magnesium cream. And I find if I've been sitting a lot during the day that my legs and my back will ache at night, and I'll need to do a few minutes of light yoga or stretching right before I hop into bed to loosen up my tight muscles; it really makes a big difference.

So, to sum up: sleep is good and quality sleep is better!

You can have a big impact on your symptoms by slowly retraining your mind and body to need less sleep during the day and to fall asleep and wake up at regular times, with plenty of deep sleep in between. Regular exercise and meditation, and changing your routine at night will help you to have a healthier sleep cycle, with plenty of quality, restorative sleep.

Your affirmation for this chapter is: *Party all day, sleep all night.*

GOLDEN NUGGETS

Here's the chapter you've all been waiting for: the one where I tell you the drugs you need to take to make you all better. The other chapters, about cutting all your favourite foods out of your life, starting regular movement, getting your attitude sorted, and the rest, are all just to make the book look thicker and to make you think you were getting value for your money!

The truth is, you can just go to any doctor, tell them you have fibromyalgia, and they'll give you a prescription for some pills that will treat all of your symptoms. Easy, right?

Nope, sorry, it's not that easy. Sorry to get your hopes up, but come on, you already knew that. You already knew that there isn't a quick fix for fibromyalgia. That's really why you bought this book.

Good news, as you've already read in the last eight chapters, there's plenty you can do to kick-start your healing. The fact is, though, you could be doing everything else right, you could do everything in this book, to the letter, but if you haven't treated what's really going on inside the body, it could all be a big fat waste of your time.

Some of the supplements I've tried have been good for more energy, better sleep, pain management, or migraines. In general, you may find that if you can add in some vitamin, mineral or herbal supplements, you can reduce your reliance on prescription pain medicine. Yes, you can get yourself some golden nuggets of happiness!

I'm not going to talk about the drugs today, except to say, do your research on what's being recommended to you and, remember, you are CEO here—if you are not comfortable with what's being offered to you, be straight with your doctor and have a discussion around your concerns.

Okay, nurse hat on now. Even if you don't need to discuss current meds, you've got to check with your doctor before starting on any pills, whether vitamins, or herbal supplements, or over-the-counter or prescription medication. Especially if you're already taking something, or have other medical conditions—it is super important before you add in any new pills or powders.

I'm not a doctor or a pharmacist, so I'm not qualified to advise anybody on what medication or supplements are right for them, but I can tell you what has worked for me.

Personally, I haven't taken any prescription medication for fibromyalgia, apart from short-term use of a migraine preventer. I tend to be very sensitive to medication and I don't want to deal with the side effects. Who needs nasty side effects when you've already got so many other symptoms going on? No, thanks!

That's not to say that side effects aren't possible with supplements, because they certainly are, and it is possible to become very sick, even with the most 'natural' of products. You need to be cautious, and that's why it's important to check in with your doctor if you want to try anything new.

I take over-the-counter pain medication, ibuprofen or paracetamol, for pain when I really need to, but that's it. However, over the years, I have found certain vitamin, mineral or herbal supplements that have worked for me. I've found that these supplements have helped my body to heal faster, and help to prevent flare-ups, without nasty side effects. When I do get flare-ups, I feel like I can knock them on the head quickly, and move on with my week.

Of all of the supplements I've tried, I'd have to say magnesium has the biggest impact on me. Magnesium is great for mood and helping your body deal with stress, and inflammation, better. It's really good for supporting your nerve health, and your whole nervous system.

Since I started taking magnesium regularly, I've had less muscle and joint pain, migraines, PMS symptoms, and period pain. If I miss magnesium for more than a day my muscles feel tighter, and I get leg cramps during the night; I feel tired more easily, and I'm a bit more irritable.

The supplements I take have magnesium amino acid chelate in them; there's a few different forms of magnesium used in supplements, but I found the others I tried upset my stomach. Starting on a higher dose of magnesium can also cause stomach upset, so I gradually increased how much I was taking per day. I now take half a gram of magnesium twice a day, and I bump that up to half a gram three times a day if I'm sick, travelling, dealing with a mini flare-up, etc.

The next supplement that's been helpful for my symptoms is vitamin B12—it's kind of like a 'little ray of sunshine' vitamin. Low levels of vitamin B12 are quite common in women with fibromyalgia, and there's a whole host of reasons for that that I won't go into, but I will say that stress and anxiety are really good at depleting the body of vitamin B12. Vitamin B12 is important for your body to make energy, and it can be a great mood booster as well. It's also good for concentration and clearing brain fog, and can help prevent digestion from getting sluggish.

Methyl cobalamin is the most active form of vitamin B12, and it is best absorbed by the body if taken in a dissolvable tablet or spray under the tongue. You can also get vitamin B12 as an intramuscular injection (needle in the bum), but that's something you need to talk to your doctor about—they'll probably want you to have a blood test first, and will then decide whether your level of B12 is low enough to warrant that method. I'd highly recommend getting a blood test to check your vitamin B12 levels before you start taking it in any form. Too much B12 in the blood can cause some icky neurological symptoms.

When I was very sick with vestibular migraines last year, and I was really struggling to look after myself, let alone my girls, my doctor and I agreed that I needed to start on a migraine preventative medication. Almost overnight I started to feel better, but I also started to feel ravenous all day long—a common side effect of the drug. At the time, I felt like I really needed to stay on the preventative medication, but I wanted to stop taking it as soon as possible, so I talked to my doctor about a vitamin and herbal supplement called Migraine Care.

I had heard that Migraine Care was a good, natural option for treating and preventing migraines, and that some neurologists had started prescribing it for their patients with chronic migraines. I knew it could take two to three months before the supplement had a real effect, so my doctor and I decided I should take the preventative medication and Migraine Care together for at least two months.

After that, I was able to gradually wean myself off the preventative medication, and still feel pretty good. If you suffer from migraines regularly, you might like to speak to your doctor about trying Migraine Care (it requires a prescription), and if you're already taking migraine preventative medication, do not stop taking it suddenly.

You might remember from Had a Gutful that if our gut isn't healthy, we're not going to feel healthy. You need to be mindful of what you're putting into your body now, but also consider that damage may have already been done, and you may need some help to heal it. Poor diet, chronic stress and antibiotic use can cause damage to the lining of your intestines, and you can end up with a condition called leaky gut.

A lot of fibromyalgia symptoms are quite similar to leaky gut symptoms, and there's talk in the scientific/medical world that leaky gut may actually lead to fibro in some way, that there's some kind of cause-and-effect relationship going on there.

I won't go into detail about leaky gut—there's so much information easily accessible on the internet—but if you have found yourself an integrative medicine doctor, they should be able to test you for leaky gut with a simple urine test that only takes a few minutes. Even if you don't have leaky gut, the more you can do to make your digestive system healthier, the better you're going to feel overall.

I take a broad spectrum probiotic every morning, and at night I drink a gut repair powder mixed with water. The powder contains glutamine, slippery elm bark, aloe vera, curcumin (the active component of turmeric), and a prebiotic—all of which have been found to be good for reducing inflammation and healing throughout the digestive system.

With the probiotic, the powder, and avoiding gluten, dairy, sugar and alcohol, I would say my guts has never been healthier!

With any of these supplements or powders it can take around two to three months before you notice any difference. After getting the go-ahead from your doctor, start with just one, so that you can see if you experience any side effects. You might find you have some mild stomach upset or your bowel habits might change when you first start something new, and often that will ease in a week or two as your body gets used to it.

Of course, if you have any nasty side effects, check in with your doctor immediately or get yourself to the hospital before you continue to take that supplement. Also, if you only try one new product at a time, you will be able to know whether it's worth continuing to take or if you're wasting your money, depending on whether or not you notice improvement in your symptoms.

Supplements can be quite expensive, so you don't want to be taking any more than you need to. If you've been taking one for three months, and have found some improvement in your symptoms, but it's not quite enough, you can then try adding in another, and again wait three months before trying another supplement. If adding in another supplement doesn't improve your symptoms after three months, then don't keep taking it—it's just money down the drain if it doesn't help you.

Now, if you started taking some supplements, exercising regularly, meditating, and sorting out your diet, and are feeling pretty good, you might be tempted to throw your drugs in the bin. I've got to put my nurse hat on again now, and warn you against that.

If you've been on medication long term, especially prescription pain meds, anti-depressants or anti-anxieties, you cannot stop taking them suddenly—you've got to wean off them slowly, under doctor's supervision. If you stop cold turkey, or reduce your dose too quickly, you're going to have some pretty nasty effects, so please have a chat with your doctor if you want to reduce your medication.

You might already have a bunch of scripts at the chemist, and go in month to month and pick up your meds, and take your meds regularly, and you might be feeling pretty good. You might be thinking, I don't need to try any of the natural supplements or the airy-fairy herbal stuff.

I think it's great if you've found something that is helping you. But there's no harm in trying supplements (as long as you check with your doctor about possible interactions with the supplements and prescription meds), and you might even see more improvement, maybe even wean off those prescription meds at some point.

Well, I've given you a lot of information in this chapter, although I really tried to keep it short and sweet, without too much science mumbo jumbo. I want to finish up with a suggestion that will hopefully help you to get the most out of this chapter—use your journal to keep a track of your symptoms as you are trying supplements.

Seeing it in black and white can help you see what is or isn't working for you. It could be as simple as: day 1 of magnesium, no change, bit of an upset tummy; day 4, think I had a bit of a better sleep last night, stomach still a bit icky, will lower the dose and see how I go; day 10, no headache today, able to remember kids' names more easily.

Your affirmation for this chapter is: *I'm going to get me the goods.*

BE THE MOTH

I'm sure you all know the saying 'like a moth to a flame'? Those ugly night-time butterflies really have a weird attraction to light, don't they? Well, it's time for you to develop the same weird attraction. Go to the light, be friends with the light. Let go of the darkness and aim for the light at the end of the tunnel. All right, that's a lot of metaphors, but hopefully you get the gist of what I'm saying? Maybe not.

Plain and simple, it's time now for you to look forward and move forward. Hang on to the belief that you will heal and that things will get better, if you just keep moving forward, towards the light at the end of the tunnel. What is your light? What is it that you are drawn to when you think about a life post recovery?

Maybe your light is finishing a uni degree, or being able to play with your kids. Maybe it's being able to stay awake past 8 p.m. so you can enjoy a date night with your hubby. Maybe it's writing a book and launching your own online business. Maybe it's just being able to get through normal, day-to-day bits and pieces without a nap. Whatever your light is, be the moth and allow yourself to form a slightly obsessive attraction to it.

Once you find your light and you've got yourself heading towards it, you'll find it's so much easier to stay on track with the whole healing process. You'll find that it will just naturally progress, because you will have your light (whatever it may be for you) in your sights, and it will be easier for your mind to focus on going forwards.

The mind is a very powerful tool in healing, but we tend to need to know what we're aiming for before we can get there. At the start of the book I spoke about the effect that your attitude, or mindset, has on your ability to recover from fibromyalgia.

Essentially, your mindset dictates where you end up. When I had my AC day, it was as though something switched on in my head, and all of a sudden I wasn't cool with accepting that for the rest of my life I would feel as crappy as I did then, and I wanted better for myself. I didn't have a book to tell me that it was possible to have the life I wanted, I just knew I deserved better. I figured, what's the harm in aiming high and giving it a go—surely I couldn't make myself feel any worse than I already did.

You know what's great about hitting rock bottom? The only way to go from there is up! I had this vision in my head of what I wanted my life to be, and I just kept heading towards it.

I had everybody saying fibromyalgia, that sucks, but you can't do much about it, just take it easy. I just kept saying, no, I want better than this. I want to be a better mum to my kids; I want to finish uni and get a job; I want to find love and live happily ever after. I didn't know if I was barking up the wrong tree, I just kept focusing in that direction—I was the moth and I wanted to get to my light.

In the end I got there, and then I wanted more, so my light changed. And now look at me—I've written a book! If I'd never had my AC day, and stopped accepting that fibromyalgia had ruined my life forever, then I never would have gotten to where I am now.

Regardless of what I was being told was possible, I believed I'd get to my light one day. If you can't let yourself believe that you'll reach yours, then you won't. You are going to continue having nasty flare-ups, and your life will continue to be dictated by your symptoms. You may make some progress, but it will be inconsistent.

It's going to take so much longer to get where you want to be, or you will fall short, if you can't allow yourself to believe it is possible to have the life that you want, and to keep your focus on your light. You need to love the light, and be drawn to the light, and you will get there. You don't need to worry about falling short of your ideal life at the end, because you'll make it happen, your attitude will get you there.

If you are a very visual person you might need to be able to see your ideal life in a concrete form, so you might like to try vision boards. When I come across phrases or pictures that I find inspirational I cut them out and stick them up somewhere in my bedroom, where I know I'll see them every day. If you're exposing yourself to images of your light every day, it will be easier for your mind to focus on where you want to get to, and how you're going to get there.

You might have been in the fibro fog for so long now that you don't even know what your light is, you don't even know what you want out of life anymore, or maybe you're scared of getting your hopes up and failing. That's okay.

For the moment, just focus on a symptom—maybe you can say my light is a life where I feel less fatigued, or my light is a life where I don't have migraines on a weekly basis. That can be enough for now. At least you will be aiming for something. Your light doesn't need to be something like finish my PhD, get married and have a bunch of kids, or solve all of the world's problems and bring about world peace.

It can be scary to have hope—with hope comes the possibility that we might be disappointed or fail—so, if all you can focus on at the moment is one symptom improving, then at least you're doing one better than accepting the status quo.

As long as you have something in mind that you want to work towards, you will move forward. Don't expect overnight miracles, and as you progress, your confidence will grow. With each success, no matter how small, you will find that you will allow yourself to hope for more, and you will find that your light becomes a more ambitious target.

This chapter is about looking forwards, so this is going to sound contradictory, but it can be a good idea, at this point, to reflect on how far you have already come. In fact, it can help renew your focus on moving forwards, which sounds really weird, but, trust me, it does.

If you can see that six months ago you were trying to get from A to B, and now you're well on your way to D, it can be very motivating. You can see that you are definitely making progress, which can be hard to see when you are in the thick of it. It can be really disheartening if you are trying so hard to do everything you can to heal, and then you get hit with a flare-up. It can feel like you are getting nowhere, and the light at the end of the tunnel can seem so very far away still.

If I even have a day now where I feel a little more fatigued than usual, I feel frustrated, and my mind will tell me that I'm never going to be free of fibromyalgia. Then I remember where I started, and a little fatigue for a day really doesn't seem so bad in comparison. So instead of feeling frustrated, I give myself a break, and focus only on what really needs to be done that day, knowing that I'll get myself back on track once the fatigue passes.

Your journal can be very useful on those days—reading through it will help you to see how far you have come, and will remind you that you are making progress.

For me, part of reflecting is feeling gratitude for all of the progress I've made with my recovery, and how much I've already accomplished. Every day I come up with at least three things that I am grateful for. At the start of your recovery, it might be something as simple as I'm grateful that today I was able to reduce my nap by 10 minutes. That's an achievement! You are already closer to your ideal life than you were yesterday, and that's something to feel grateful for. Maybe in a few months you might feel grateful that you were able to cook a nutritious meal for your family, and you could sit at the table to eat it with them.

Appreciate every little step you take towards your light, because each step is necessary and important. Just by buying this book and actually reading it, you have allowed yourself to hope that a better life may be possible for you, and you have taken a step forward. Go you! Be careful of expecting too much too soon, and pushing yourself to get somewhere before your body is ready.

Your affirmation for this chapter is: *I am the moth. I love the light at the end of the tunnel. I'm weirdly drawn to it.*

BABY STEPS

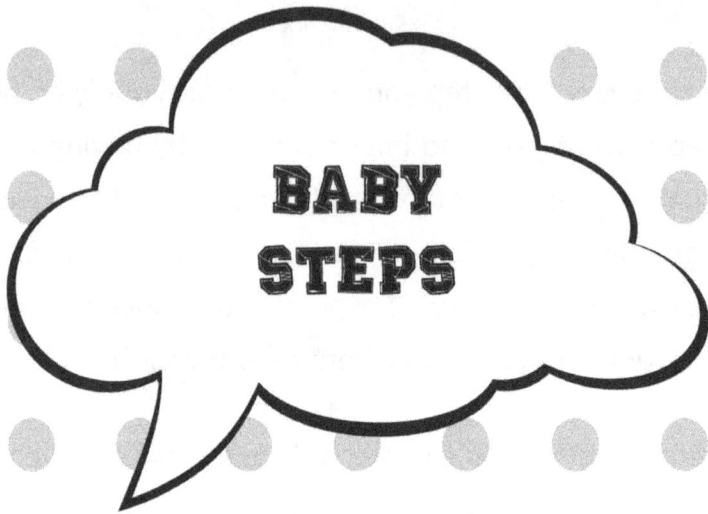

Like a baby learning to walk, your first steps forward are going to be unsteady, and it will be frustratingly difficult to make any progress at all. You may give up trying for a while and go back to commando crawling, but eventually you'll become surer-footed and will suddenly be moving forwards at a pace that will surprise you and everyone around you.

Healing your body and reclaiming your life isn't going to happen in a hurry; it's going to take time and a marathon effort to get there. But if you focus on one baby step at a time, you will get there.

If you're keeping yourself to baby steps, and realistic goals, you'll have more wins. Yay! Who doesn't like winning? Even the smallest win is better than no win at all—every win, no matter how insignificant it may seem, will help you stay motivated, and at the end of the day, any progress is better than no progress. Right?

Breaking down the whole recovery process into more manageable steps will make it seem much less overwhelming for you, and you will be more likely to achieve, and to keep going until you get to your light at the end of the tunnel.

When I first started reclaiming my life from fibromyalgia, my first goal was simply to have enough energy left over after feeding my kids to be able to sit up to eat my own dinner, every night. Sounds like a pretty small goal, right? At the time, it was actually something that was quite difficult for me—it would take every ounce of energy that I had just to cook my kids dinner (and we're not talking three courses of gourmet food or anything close to it!), and by the time I fed them and got them sorted for bed I would be so absolutely exhausted that I didn't even have the energy to sit up and eat, I would just drag myself off to bed.

Right now, it just seems like such a small achievement, but at the time it was massive, and, more importantly, it was the very first baby step of many. You have to crawl before you can run, right?

While it's important to aim for your light—the life you want for yourself—if you try to get to it too quickly, you will likely find yourself slipping backwards, and you really don't want that. You want to be making progress, consistent progress, as much as possible, but you need to try to avoid triggering flare-ups at the same time. Not only will you have to waste time recovering from each flare-up—possibly holding up your progress by days each time—your confidence will take a hit each time.

Each time your confidence is hit by a flare-up, it will be slightly harder to keep your attitude in check. Do you remember from the first chapter (Rainbows and Lollipops) how important your attitude is? Remember that if your attitude isn't right, you're just wasting your time trying anything? Reread it now if you don't remember!

You have got to work in baby steps, and not a bunch of baby steps at once. Just start with one or two baby steps at a time, and give yourself a real chance to have those wins before you even think about trying to run. When your confidence is low, it's much less painful to fall if you're only trying to take a couple of tentative baby steps, than if you try to go from standing to running.

Did you learn how to skate? Remember being taught to take little steps with the skates on first? I do. When I taught my girls to skate, I taught them the same way I was taught. They did the little steps for ages, holding on to my hands. Then they started pushing their feet out a little more with each step, still hanging on to my hands. Then they did that while gripping on to the low wall around the rink, and I would just stay nearby in case they needed me.

Eventually, they started letting go of the wall more and more, and doing more of a skate rather than steps. I barely remember seeing them fall over at all, at least not while they were learning. On the other hand, I would see other little kids at the rink who would try to go from skates on to flying around the rink in one session. Boy, were they scary to watch! They would fall over so much I don't know how the place didn't run out of ice packs!

It's all well and good to want to strap your skates on and start speed skating your way to the life that you want, but chances are you're a beginner when it comes to recovering from fibro, and you're going to need to take your time, and start with little steps first. Once you've got your first goal (or two) in your head, it's good to have a game plan for how you're going to progress to your light at the end of the tunnel, but you need to be flexible.

Check in with yourself regularly about where you are at, and what your next step is going to be. Ask yourself is this really achievable for me at the moment, or is there a step I need to take before I can get to that? Write your thoughts in your journal and really be mindful of whether you are taking nice steady steps forward, or if you are trying to push too hard too fast.

You have to be reasonable and flexible with your time frames. It's all well and good to say I want to go from the couch to running a marathon in a month—that's certainly aiming high—but that may not be a reasonable expectation for your body, even if you are doing everything right. If you push yourself to run that marathon before your body is ready, you may end up back where you started.

It's like trying to build the brick walls of a house before the foundation has become hard—the walls will crack and fall apart, the foundation will be ruined, and the builders would have to start from scratch all over again.

If you're a high achiever like me, there will be days when you feel frustrated with your progress, and you'll feel like you need to be pushing yourself harder, aiming higher, expecting more of yourself. You will need to remind yourself that the harder you push the more likely you are to go backwards, and going backwards will only make you feel pissed off!

If it takes you two years of consistent progress before you are able to run a marathon, would that make it any less of an achievement? If you could run that whole marathon and recover within a few days, wouldn't that be better than pushing yourself to the brink for a month, not being able to finish the marathon, and then taking months before you get back to feeling like you did before you attempted the marathon?

When you are feeling frustrated with taking baby steps, and feeling like you aren't progressing fast enough, go back to your vision board, your symptoms diary, and your gratitude and reflection writing in your journal. Remind yourself that you are having wins, and you are achieving. I guarantee you will feel less frustrated.

You're going to have days when you feel overwhelmed with how far you still have to go, and how many steps are still ahead of you. You will think there's so many things that I want to work on—I need to fix my sleep, I want to feel less fatigued, I have to exercise more, I've got to stop eating sugar ... I just don't know what to work on first, and I can't see that I'm ever going to have it all sorted. I've been there, and not just with my recovery from fibromyalgia.

I find if I really want to tackle something, like cleaning the house, for example, I need to have some kind of plan of attack in mind. If I don't, I feel overwhelmed with how much I have to get done, so I procrastinate to avoid feeling overwhelmed, and then nothing gets done!

Consider this book your plan of attack. Start with the first chapter (Rainbows and Lollipops), pick a date for your AC day, and decide what steps you need to take to get your attitude sorted. When you've done all you think you can for the first chapter, move on to the second chapter (Who's in Charge?), and do the steps that need to be done for that chapter, and so on. Before too long, you'll find that taking one step naturally leads you to take the next one and the next.

Or if you want to approach fibromyalgia in a different way, pick the chapter you want to start with and go from there. If you don't want to follow the order of chapters as I've written them, I'd still recommend starting with Rainbows and Lollipops to give yourself the best chance of success.

From time to time you will get to a point where you think I've been trying to get to the next step for ages and I just seem stuck where I am. There will be some steps that will be bloody hard, and will take longer to achieve. By the same token, at some steps you will surprise yourself, and smash them out straight up. Those wins will keep you going, and will help you to be patient when you feel stuck. Sometimes a *small*—with lots of emphasis on the word *small*—push, or a change in focus can make a big difference, without doing yourself harm.

When you do feel stuck, have a look at what you're doing and see if there's anything at all you can tweak—is there something in your diet that you can look at changing? Can you increase your movement by a minute? Can you cut an extra five minutes from your daytime sleep?

If you tweak a little and trigger a bit of a flare-up (although that's unlikely if you've only pushed a little), accept that you're not ready to move on to the next step, and that's okay. Focus on getting back to where you are comfortable, and just maintain it for a while. Sit on your hands and take the time to think about how much you've already achieved. Or, you can try a shift in focus and you may find that gets you to the next step.

For example, if you've been able to march on the spot for five minutes, for three days a week, for a few weeks, without your fatigue or muscle pain feeling worse, your next step might be to march on the spot for five minutes, four days a week. When it comes to the first week, you can only manage a minute of marching on the fourth day before you feel you have to stop, and the same thing happens again the next week. The following week, you could go back to just the three days, but start using an app to make sure you are drinking enough water every day, and after doing that for two or three weeks you can try marching on the spot for the fourth day again. A small tweak, or a slight change in focus can make a big difference.

Remember, baby steps are the key to consistently moving forward, with little to no time wasted going backwards in your recovery. Have a rough idea of the baby steps you need to take, and use this book as a guide for the order of the steps.

There will be times when you feel frustrated with what seems like slow progress, but reflecting on where you have come from can remind you that any progress is better than no progress. You will need to be patient with your body, and if you get stuck on a step, a little tweaking or a change in focus can get you moving again.

Your affirmation for this chapter is: *One small step for them is one giant leap for me.*

CLEANING FANS

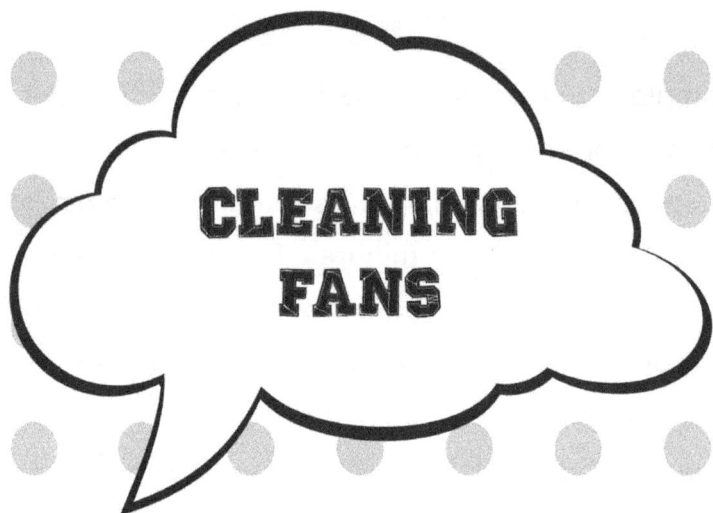

As I'm expecting most of the readers of this book to be adults who have been doing life for a while I'm going to assume that you all know and accept that sometimes in life the proverbial will hit the fan. It's not always about rainbows and lollipops, after all.

It's all well and good to act on everything you read in this book and be the perfect case study for healing from fibromyalgia (just like I am, of course). You could even work one on one with a nurse health coach (hint hint, nudge nudge) to keep you on track and feeling motivated.

However, there will be times when you are under far more emotional and physical stress than your body can handle, and chances are you'll be rewarded with a flare-up. The reality is you may always have to deal with flare-ups, but flare-ups don't mean starting from scratch.

Lucky for you, you still have this book and if you follow through with everything I've been talking about for the past 11 chapters, your flare-ups will be much less severe, much less frequent, you'll be able to manage them a lot better and you will bounce back to where you were quicker each time.

When your fans get covered in you know what, you've just got to clean them off and remember that you are in charge of your health. You are more resilient than you think you are. After all, you've read most of this book now.

Be kind to yourself. Tweak where you feel you need to, or do what you need to get through the flare-up—maybe nap a little more, take a break from cooking gourmet meals for the family for a while—then pick yourself up and keep taking baby steps towards your friend, the light.

The less pressure that you put on yourself, the less severe your flare-ups are going to be, and you'll be able to nip them in the bud and bounce back faster. If you are patient with your body and accept that some days are going to be crappy, you're more likely to stay on track and make solid progress, and you'll build endurance each time.

It's about accepting that there's only so much that we can control in our lives. While you can do everything possible to make yourself well, to heal yourself, and to get to the life that you want, there are going to be days when you're going to get knocked down. In time, though, you will find that you will be able to get back up and recover quicker.

I was actually really sick earlier last year and I really don't get sick much at all. This one kind of came out of the blue, and it threw me for six. It started as a bit of a head cold, but within days I had really severe vertigo, then I started having trouble with my balance and coordination, my vision was playing tricks on me, and I had this horrible feeling of being completely disconnected from my limbs. I had an MRI and blood tests, and thankfully everything came back clear, but my doctor didn't know what was wrong with me, and so there wasn't much he could do to help me feel better.

For the first time in a really long time I was bedridden, and I couldn't do the things that I needed to do each day. I had to rely on family to help me out with my girls. I had to stop working at the GP clinic where I was working as a nurse, and I had to go back to focusing on my health, resting, and looking after myself.

If it had been 18 months to two years ago, I would have been really frustrated and upset with myself that I couldn't just pick myself up and move on with life. Instead, I accepted that it was temporary, that it would pass, and that it didn't mean that I was going back to where I started from. I knew it didn't mean that everything I'd done in the last few years for my health had been a waste of time, or that I needed to question everything that I was doing.

I knew all it meant was that I had probably picked up some random virus, and I needed to listen to my body and give it what it needed—rest. After a few weeks I was diagnosed with vestibular migraines, which must have been triggered by the head cold I had. I started on the migraine preventer medication and supplement that I wrote about in Golden Nuggets. Even so, it took me about three months to fully recover back to where I was before I got that head cold. Three months might sound like a long time, but when I think about how sick I really was, it seems kind of impressive that it only took me that long to recover.

I could have thrown my hands up and thought, what's the point— I've worked so hard to get to this really amazing point where I feel so great, but then I get knocked down, big time. What's the point? The point is, apart from that time, for the last two or three years I've barely had more than a bit of leg or back pain, a day here or there when I felt tired (but who doesn't?) and the odd headache. I don't even know if they really classify as fibromyalgia symptoms anymore; I mean, most people without fibro would have the odd headache or backache.

Regardless, I pay attention to my body, and because I know that flare-ups are still a possibility, I don't ignore any niggles. Prevention is better than cure, as the saying goes, and I don't want to have to deal with pulling myself out of a flare-up if I can help it.

If my back aches I'll stretch more, if my head aches I'll drink more water or rest more, if my legs are sore I'll have a hot bath and then rub magnesium cream into my muscles. I give my body what I think it needs, and I get myself back on track. Usually, within 6 – 12 hours my 'symptoms' are gone.

Can you imagine getting to the point where you have enough faith in your body that no matter what gets thrown your way, you will get through it? That you will be able to pick yourself up and get on with your life even quicker than you ever thought you could, and each time it would be quicker and easier than the last?

I can tell you, it's a wonderful feeling. But if you can't get your head around the fact that flare-ups will happen, and that life is going to throw all sorts of crap your way, then you are really going to struggle to get there.

Early on, I would get to the point where I was seeing some real progress and feeling good about myself, and then I would crash and burn. I'd think, what's the point, and I'd get all 'woe is me', 'life is so unfair', 'why do bad things always happen to me?' and I'd give up trying.

It would take me weeks before I'd even think about trying to take baby steps again. I wasted so much time going backwards or just not trying. We humans really hate to fail, don't we? But what if you thought of flare-ups not as signs of failure, but just as bumps in the road?

We're all going to have low days when we feel like we're getting nowhere. To get you through those days, try writing a letter to yourself on a day when you're feeling really good. In the letter remind yourself that flare-ups are only temporary, that you are in fact making progress, and you feel amazing because you are doing everything that you can do to get to the life that you want. Tell yourself how you have progressed (e.g. I'm only napping for about 10 minutes now, or I've been sugar free for six weeks and I've got so much more energy), and that you will be feeling good again in no time.

It's hard in the moments of feeling like rubbish to remember that you are making progress, that you are getting closer to the life that you want, but reading it in black and white makes it a lot easier for our minds to believe.

Something that I wish I had known about and accessed in the early days is a health coach. A health coach would have kept me motivated and moving forwards. It would have been handy to have somebody who I could turn to during the flare-ups, and those days when I was ready to give up—somebody who would say, this is just temporary, you are going to get through this, you are going to get back to where you were and you will one day have the life that you want.

If you can't afford a health coach at the moment, maybe a family member or friend could be that person for you. Sometimes, even when we logically know something is true in our own minds, we don't really believe it until we hear somebody else say it.

Hopefully this book will also be like a printed version of a health coach for you: something that you can pick up on the rough days and by seeing that there's pages and pages of options and possibilities for healing yourself, feel more hopeful and ready to pick yourself up off the floor.

You can also think about joining fibromyalgia support pages and my Facebook group page, Positively FibromyAWESOME!, and get support from others to boost you up and help you get back on track when you're feeling ready to give up.

So, get some contingency plans in place for when your fans get covered—write yourself a letter, find a health coach or a loved one who can keep you motivated. Above all else, go easy on yourself, and expect that life will throw curve balls your way on occasion.

At the end of the day, you need to remember that flare-ups are temporary, and you are a lot more resilient than you think. It might not feel like it on the really bad days, but just know that you are. You are a strong woman, and you will claw your life back from fibromyalgia, one baby step at a time.

Your affirmation for this chapter is: *When poo hits the fan, I can clean it off and move on.*

AFTERWORD

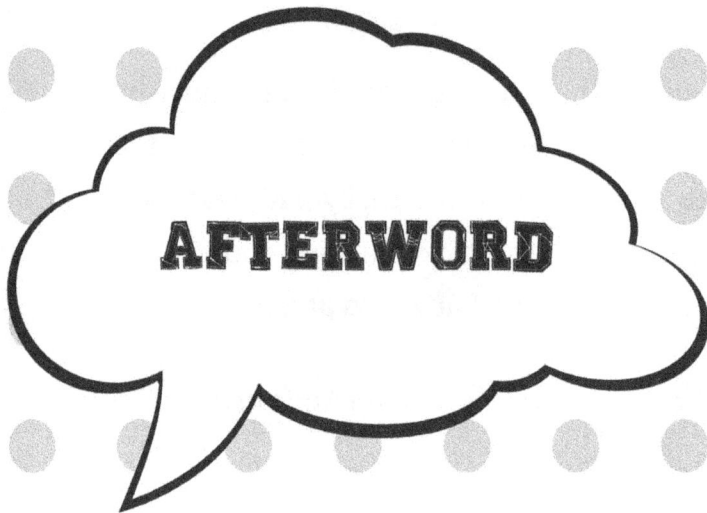

Wow! You finished this book! Congratulations! You read the whole book, with fatigue, foggy head, pain and crappy sleep cycles, and you're here, you are at the end of the book! Round of applause for you! You've already achieved something!

You might remember that I suggested in the first chapter that you don't try to implement too much when you first read through this book, and that you should just take your time and get to know my story, and understand where I started, and how I got to where I am now.

If this is the first time that you've read through this book, hopefully you can appreciate that my health and my life were pretty crappy when I first decided to start trying to heal myself.

Where I started is probably very similar to where you are now, or where you started from. If you got nothing else from reading this book for the first time, I hope you at least have some hope now. I hope that you now know that you do have options, and that you do not have to give up your whole life to fibromyalgia. I hope that you believe that you can get your life back, and maybe even go on to have an even healthier, better life than you had before.

If this is your first time reading FibromyAWESOME, just take some time to process all of the information, and then when you're ready, start the book again, and take it one chapter at a time. I'd recommend going through each chapter in order; I've written it in an order I feel would work best in terms of long-term recovery.

Take your time, aim for steady progress, and don't feel bad if you can't do everything all in one smooth process. If you make one adjustment, and then don't come back for a couple of months, that's okay—it's not about how quickly you get the results, it's about maintaining long-term results. Any progress is good progress, remember!

This book is a bit of a condensed guide to how I healed myself from fibro, and I wrote it so that it would be easy to read. There's so much more detail that I could go into for most of the chapters, but I wanted everyone to be able to kick-start their own recovery without having to take a hammer to their piggy banks.

If you'd like to take your recovery and your health to the next level, but aren't sure how to go about it, please check out my offers at the back of this book, and on my website ultimateyoubyyou.com.

At the moment, remember to focus on taking those baby steps one at a time, and make sure you've got your fist-pump crew around you to keep you supported and to encourage you the whole way.

Stay hopeful, and be kind to yourself along the way—there is no such thing as a perfect recovery!

Spread the word that there is hope, and there are options for recovery, and support others who may be thinking about kick-starting their own recovery, or who may have already started.

I encourage all of you to reach out on social media and in forums for support, and please reach out to me too! I'd love to know what you think of the book, and how your recovery is going, so please get in touch with me via my email ultimateyoubyyou.com and my Facebook page: facebook.com/ultimateyoubyyou.

Okay, so you are nearly at the end of this book, and there are not a lot of pages left, and you might be thinking, well, hang on, when is she going to tell me how to cure fibromyalgia? I've nearly finished reading this awesome book, this must be the part where she says that she's completely cured from fibromyalgia.

Sorry, not cured here. Well, not yet anyway! Well I don't really think about it like that anyway. Whether I still fit the diagnostic criteria for fibromyalgia or not, it doesn't matter—it's nothing more than a label. At the end of the day, if the worst I have to deal with is a bit of leg pain or backache, or the odd headache or bit of fatigue, then I'm doing very well, whether I have fibro or not. I mean, who doesn't get a niggly ache now and then, or the occasional headache?

You might not have noticed, but I've never actually used the word cure in terms of fibromyalgia. This book has been about my experiences recovering from fibromyalgia, and being able to heal from fibromyalgia so that I can live the life that I want.

Fibromyalgia may always be a part of our lives. That does not mean that we have to accept a life spent in pain on the couch, and I really, really hope that you believe that now. I hope that by sharing my story, you now believe that it is possible for you to live the life that you want, with or without fibromyalgia.

Give yourself a big pat on the back now, because you've finished this book! You are going to change your life. You are going to go get it done. You are going to go for the light and be drawn to the light. I am so excited for you! I wish you all the very, very best in health and in life.

Now go be FibromyAWESOME!

ABOUT THE AUTHOR

Melanie spent much of her carefree childhood in the remote Queensland mining town of Mt. Isa. After tragically losing her mum to leukaemia at the age of 16, Melanie completed her senior years of high school in Brisbane, and went on to graduate from university with an Applied Science degree in animal studies. Melanie had hopes of one day going on to achieve her childhood dream of becoming a veterinarian. Instead, what followed was a short-lived marriage, and two beautiful daughters, Rhiannon and Isobel.

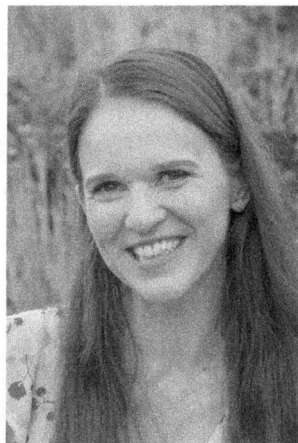

At the age of 30—divorced and struggling to get by as a single mum to her young girls—Melanie enrolled in a nursing degree.

For five years, her strong desire to help others kept her going, as she juggled day-to-day life and university studies. During that time, Rhiannon was diagnosed with the rare genetic disorder Williams Syndrome, and needed countless hours of therapy each week, as well as regular appointments with specialist doctors.

At the same time, Melanie was diagnosed with the debilitating condition fibromyalgia—a condition characterised by chronic fatigue, muscle pain, joint aches, migraines, trouble concentrating, memory problems and insomnia. Despite all of this, Melanie graduated nursing with distinction—a testament to her grit and determination.

Melanie's doctors had told her that there wasn't much they could do for fibromyalgia, and she would just have to learn to live with the symptoms. After deciding one day (the day she now calls her AC, or Attitude Change, day) that she wasn't going to accept that the rest of her life would be dictated by fibromyalgia— a life spent lying on the couch, exhausted, while her children watched TV—Melanie set about healing herself, and getting her life back from fibromyalgia.

Slowly but surely, Melanie began to feel better, and over a few years her symptoms improved dramatically. After experiencing burnout working shiftwork as a nurse, Melanie decided her focus needed to be on her health and wellbeing, and her daughters.

Becoming an author was never in Melanie's life plan, but when a friend asked her to write some tips for a friend of hers who had recently been diagnosed with fibromyalgia, the idea of sharing her knowledge through a book suddenly made sense.

Melanie's greatest wish is that others don't have to suffer the debilitating symptoms of fibromyalgia for years like she did. Melanie also understands there are many more women who may not have a chronic condition, such as fibromyalgia, but who are worn out, overworked, always putting themselves last, and running on empty most days.

Believing that all of these women are in need of someone who can guide and motivate them to a healthier, happier life, Melanie decided she could help even more women as a nurse health coach—and her health coaching business, Mello Motivation (re-launched in March 2020 as Ultimate You By You; ultimateyoubyyou.com), was born.

Melanie now lives in Townsville, in tropical north Queensland, with her daughters Rhiannon, 12, and Isobel, 10 and her husband Sean, and his daughter, Ally, 14. She spends her days wearing her many hats: mum, wife, author, health coach, nurse and blogger—and she rarely needs a daytime nap anymore!

Amazing Fibro Fighting Smoothie Powder Recipe

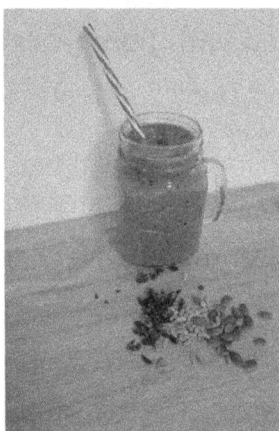

A blend of super foods and all-natural ingredients known for their anti-inflammatory and fatigue-busting properties, Melanie's amazing Fibro Fighting Smoothie Powder will give you a daily energy boost and fuel the healing process.

All ingredients in the Fibro Fighting Smoothie Powder have been scientifically shown to increase energy levels, and/or reduce inflammation and pain throughout the body, in addition to improving general health, without the possible damaging complications of artificial protein smoothie powders.

Melanie drinks a Fibro Fighting Smoothie every day for a quick and simple hit of plant-based protein, vitamins, minerals and healthy fats.

Melanie would like you to take advantage of the amazing benefits of her Fibro Fighting Smoothie Powder!

FREE!

Head to ultimateyoubyyou.com now and sign up to the Ultimate You By You subscriber list to receive the amazing Fibro Fighting Smoothie Powder recipe!

FREE!

30-Minute Fibro-Up My Life Mentoring Session

Feeling overwhelmed?

Sick and tired of feeling sick and tired?

Hoping for a healthier and happier life?

Read the book, but still not sure where to start?

<u>Available only to valued readers of FibromyAWESOME</u>

You get:

- ✓ 30-minute one-on-one mentoring session with FibromyAWESOME author, and nurse health coach, Melanie O'Shea, founder of Mello Motivation (now known as Ultimate You By You)

- ✓ Five ways you can immediately improve your health with ease

- ✓ **Tips and suggestions to implement these five strategies** into your life

You pay: **Nothing!**

Email <u>hello@ultimateyoubyyou.com</u> with the subject line 'I'm ready to start improving my health today!' to take advantage of this special offer.

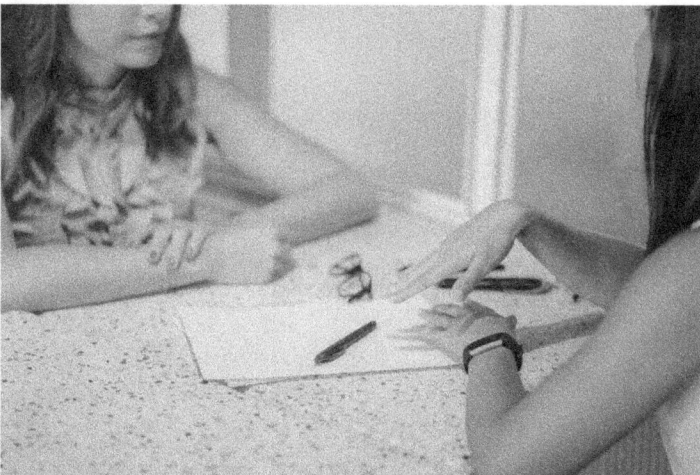

Nurse Health Coaching

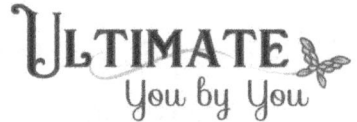

ULTIMATE
You by You

Ultimate You By You has a health coaching program for everyone, from the budget conscious and those who are not quite ready to commit, to those who are ready to transform their lives and dive in headfirst.

All programs include regular one-on-one health coaching sessions with a health coach via phone or Zoom, unlimited email support and a bunch of goodies.

Ultimate You By You's health coaching programs are personally created by Melanie, a degree-educated nurse, and are tailored to your individual needs and goals.

Our programs are great for:
- ✓ Giving your health journey a kick-start
- ✓ Setting realistic goals
- ✓ Addressing the roadblocks holding you back
- ✓ Keeping you accountable
- ✓ Increasing your chances of success
- ✓ Supporting and motivating you to a happier, healthier life!

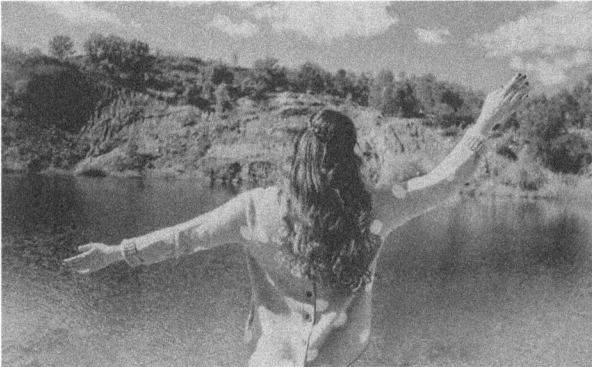

Email hello@ultimateyoubyyou.com with the subject line
'I want in on a program!'
to receive more information about
Ultimate You By You health coaching programs and
receive a **20% discount** when you sign up.

www.ingramcontent.com/pod-product-compliance
Lightning Source LLC
Chambersburg PA
CBHW031128020426
42333CB00012B/281